♡

10/00

To Sheri —

Thank you for bring the loving maternal presence that you are in so many young lives.

With love, light

your daughter

&

Lauren

Zuzu's Petals

Zuzu's Petals

A True Story of Second Chances

Lauren Ward Larsen

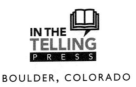

IN THE
TELLING
PRESS

BOULDER, COLORADO

Grateful acknowledgment is made to the following individuals for permission to quote previously copyrighted works: Glen Hansard for lyrics to "Falling Slowly," music and lyrics by Glen Hansard and Marketa Irglova, Copyright © 2006 The Swell Season; Chris Tomasino, on behalf of the author, for excerpt from *Simple Abundance: A Daybook of Comfort and Joy,* by Sarah Ban Breathnach, Copyright © 1995; Dave Woods for lyrics to "Side by Side," music and lyrics by Harry Woods, Original copyright © 1927, Callicoon Music.

Library of Congress Control Number: 2010936392
ISBN: 978-0-9829907-0-4

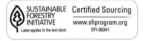

SUSTAINABLE FORESTRY INITIATIVE   Certified Sourcing
Label applies to the text stock   www.sfiprogram.org   SFI-00341

For information about special discounts on bulk purchases, please contact ZuzusPetals@InTheTelling.com. Additional discounts are available to nonprofit organizations.

A portion of both Author's and Publisher's proceeds will be donated to related charitable causes.

Book design by Gary Head

FIRST EDITION
10 9 8 7 6 5 4 3 2
Printed in the United States of America

For HB —

Fee, fi, fo, fum.
Side by side 'til the day we're numb.

INTRODUCTION

SHORTLY AFTER I MOVED TO BOULDER, Colorado, my mother stopped by my home and handed me a thick document. Across the top and in all caps it read *LAUREN'S LOG*.

"What's this?" I asked.

"It's what happened," she said.

I thumbed through page after page to see that everything she'd written in her blue notebook during the worst two months of my life was now typed up and organized, each separate date an underlined heading. Single-spaced, the pages totaled forty-seven.

"Forty-seven pages?" I asked, incredulous.

"You have no idea," Mom said. "Hell, you weren't really there half the time!" She laughed at her own joke and left to resume her morning errands.

By then, I was getting used to these whirlwind visits from Mom. Rarely a day passed that she didn't stop by to give me an interesting article she'd cut out for me or to pick up an empty Tupperware container that had held the soup she'd dropped off two days earlier. I thought the frequency of her visits was tied to the excitement of finally having one of her four grown children living in the same neighborhood, let alone in the same time zone. Today, however, I believe these visits were Mom's way of reassuring herself that the nightmare was over—that her youngest child, the one who would've been voted Most Likely to Laugh in the Face of Adversity, was still alive, and indeed laughing again.

I stood alone in my kitchen staring at Lauren's Log, my head buzzing. I'd been told that Mom had taken copious notes and collected scraps of paper with others' notes during what I now refer to simply as "the train wreck," but I was taken aback by the abruptness of actually receiving them. Over the past six months anecdotes had been doled out—gradually and tentatively—by those who'd been with me as I lay unconscious and unlikely to live, or as I screamed from physical pain so great I wanted only to die. As if putting together a jigsaw puzzle with no photo on the box to guide me, I'd taken each detail, each story, and figured out where it fit into the larger picture that was unfolding, the richness and depth of the scene not yet taking shape. I sensed that in my hands I held fistfuls of additional puzzle pieces. I tucked the document under my right arm and climbed the stairs of my new home, clutching the railing with both hands to pull the weight of my body up each step, slowly and one at a time. Reaching the second floor, I paused to catch my breath, then wobbled precariously to the overstuffed chair in my home office and sat, exhausted.

I began to read, and ten pages in I was choking back tears for these people: the baby, the husband, the new mom. *Oh my god, oh my god,* I said under my breath over and over and over again. I felt like I was watching a movie and was suddenly transposed from the audience to the screen. *Holy cow, this is me!* I remember thinking, as if discovering this fact for the first time.

I had no idea how unprepared I was to look back, naïvely believing that because I was alive and breathing and moving more each day, I was healing. I had no idea that the wounds to my psyche were far greater than the wounds to my body, that the true healing hadn't even begun.

Lauren's Log helped fill in more details, but the bigger picture revealing purpose and meaning wouldn't emerge until I began to write about it, presumably to give encouragement to others in similar situations. With ten years of hindsight, I now know that I wrote *Zuzu's Petals* for me, and in so doing gave myself the final piece of the puzzle.

Part One

~

*I knew if I were drowning, you'd try to save me.
And that's how I saved you.*

—CLARENCE ODDBODY, *It's a Wonderful Life*

I

Roses. He brought me roses. It's the middle of the afternoon, a workday no less, and my husband's six-foot-four frame fills the doorway to the guest bedroom, a bouquet of roses in hand. Still drowsy from my nap, I take a few moments to soak in his presence—the recently purchased suit that accentuates his broad shoulders and that early dusting of gray across his hairline. *Damn, he's handsome,* I think.

His smile fades, giving way to that wrinkled forehead he gets when he's concerned about one of the women in his life. When his mother broke her back. When his sister was diagnosed with multiple sclerosis. Now.

"You look awful," he says, crossing the room toward me as I lie on the bed.

"Thanks," I say. "You look like shit yourself."

He ignores my Jersey Girl shtick and sets the roses on the desk we plan to replace with the crib next week. With almost a month until the due date, we'd felt no need to rush the transformation of my office into a nursery.

I shift the weight of my body, pushing our standard poodle, Spike, off the bed with my foot. Jeff leans down and touches my bare leg. His hand recoils, touches again.

"Feels hot. Like you're sunburned," he says.

"Hmm," I say, feigning interest but wanting only to go back to sleep.

"We should go to the doctor's."

"I was just there three days ago. Everything was fine."

"Then I want to call them. At least check in."

He leaves the room and in the distance I hear the muffled sound of his voice answering questions over the phone. Minutes later he returns.

"We're going to the doctor's office. They said it's probably nothing, but they want to check your blood pressure to be sure."

"At least let me grab a quick shower and brush my teeth first," I say, but when I try to get out of bed I realize I'm too lethargic to do either. And that's when a small doubt bubbles up from deep within, breaking the smooth surface of smug certainty that has cloaked my pregnancy for eight months. What if things *aren't* okay?

I ignore my misgivings and ask Jeff to bring me something to wear. He returns carrying a baggy maternity frock and slippers—the only shoes that still fit on my sausage feet—then he helps me get dressed. Holding my arm, he guides me toward the door, but the sense that I'm forgetting something makes me look back over my shoulder.

"The roses," I say. "They need water."

"I'll get it later," he says. "When we get home."

There's an old expression: *We plan, God laughs.*

I've always been a planner, and my daughter's impending arrival has not escaped my need to control the process. My birth plan is simple: no IVs, no epidurals, no surgeons. When the time comes, I want a birthing chair, a CD of ocean sounds, and lots of deep purple helium balloons to go with the *Welcome to Earth, Clare!* sign my girlfriends and I made at the baby shower two weeks ago. As soon as I go into labor, Jeff will call my sister-in-law Dede, and she'll take the next flight from Orange County to San Francisco and meet us at the hospital. In the birthing room I'll appear calm and confident, some of which will be faked. Pacing the floor, I'll crack inappropriate jokes between sharp jabs of pain, my overuse of profanity fully excusable under the circumstances. Jeff will get nervous as each wave of labor registers on my face, but Dede, having given birth three times, will reassure him that everything's fine. Once the baby is delivered, Dede will call Liz, one of my closest gal pals, and she'll begin spreading the word of Clare's arrival to our friends and family members on the telephone list. *Mother and baby are both doing great*, I imagine Liz saying. *Damn, she's a long one*, she'll add about Clare. Those on the other end of the phone will laugh. *Of course she's a long one*, they'll say. *She's got two giants for parents!*

We arrive at my obstetrician's office, and with greater expediency than I've come to expect during prenatal visits, I'm shuffled into an examination room for a blood pressure check, then to a small bathroom for a urine sample, then back to the examination room, where my doctor tells me that my baby girl is "in distress," that I seem to have developed preeclampsia.

Pre-uh-what? I can't even spell the word, let alone tell you what it means. But apparently I've got it. And it's killing my baby, so she must be delivered immediately.

My obstetrician orders a wheelchair and before I can comprehend that my daughter's birth is happening in fast-forward, a nurse pushes me outside, across the street, into the hospital, and up to the Labor & Delivery Unit. Taking long strides, my husband keeps pace beside me. With all my carefully crafted birth plans being superseded by the urgency of the situation, Jeff and I offer one another weak consolations. We cling to what our instructor said repeatedly during the all-day birthing class we attended last month. *Your goal should be: healthy mom, healthy baby. How you get there doesn't matter.* I adopt a façade of acceptance about the impending cesarean-section surgery, but beneath all the bravado I'm terrified. If there's no reason to worry, as everyone keeps suggesting, why is everything happening so quickly? Could this preeclampsia thing actually kill my baby? I don't dare express my concerns. If I ignore them, they can't come to pass, can they? I pretend that all is well and allow my increasing exhaustion to numb my fears.

After an accelerated check-in process, I'm wheeled into a private room, where a nurse pierces both arms, my right hand, and one of my feet, but is unable to tap a vein for a blood draw. Preeclampsia, she tells me, is a common pregnancy-related condition characterized by high blood pressure and protein in the urine, and it often causes swelling beyond what is normal during pregnancy. My body now seems to be inflating by the minute. No blood sample, no epidural. And if I can't have an epidural, I'll have to go under general anesthesia, which means Jeff won't be allowed in the operating room. And I want—no, *need*—him with me.

"Please try again," I plead.

"We will," she says. "But right now we have to get you to the OR." She tells my husband to stick around, that she'll come get him if it turns out he can be present for the C-section. Jeff kisses me goodbye, and two people in blue sterile garb wheel my gurney into the hallway toward double doors that separate the surgical wing from the rest of the Labor & Delivery Unit. Inside the operating room, another nurse slaps the fleshy insides of my arms in search of a visible vein. After two tries she is successful, and blood is drawn and tested on the spot. Cleared for an epidural, I hear someone say: "Find the husband."

Two nurses press against either side of my body, holding me upright as I sit on a cold steel surgical table, a hospital gown loosely draping my front, my backside exposed. They keep a firm grip on each of my arms, like bouncers expecting a struggle from the tavern drunk who's being ejected for unruliness. I hear the words *hold still* and *small pinch*, and I immediately understand why the nurses are squeezing me so tightly.

"AHHH!" I yell, as the epidural needle is inserted into my lower spine.

"Got it," says a voice behind me.

"Small pinch, my ass," I say, trying my best to disguise the pain with sarcasm.

"Just a couple more minutes and you won't feel a thing," says the obstetrician.

I look around the sterile room with its gray linoleum floor and muted blue tile walls. The overhead lighting casts a bright glare off all the stainless steel: steel tables, steel carts, steel instruments.

"How do you feel?" asks a nurse.

How do I feel? I feel panicked and frightened by what's happening. I feel like crying. I feel like I'm losing control, and I'm *not* a woman who loses control.

"I'm good," I say. "Where's Jeff? I don't want to do this without him."

"Don't worry," she says. "We'll find him."

The bouncer nurses lower me onto my back, carefully rotating my body lengthwise as someone else lifts my legs onto the table. Although there's a plastic tube lodged in my spine, I feel nothing as I lie on top of it. Not my back, not my belly, not my legs. A nurse eases my arms into Velcro restraints and secures them to thin boards jutting out from the operating table.

"Comfortable?" she asks.

"Yes, thanks." Then, "Where's Jeff?"

"We're still trying to find him."

Despite a consistent show of confidence throughout my pregnancy, I cannot do this part without him. I don't know why I'm so anxious, and perhaps I don't want to know why, don't want to consider the possibilities that are anything but positive. I just know I need Jeff to be here.

A short blue drape is hung at my chest, blocking my view of the surgical opening through which my baby will enter the world. A lamp is positioned two or three feet over my body and I'm startled by its brightness.

"We've got to begin," says a voice from beyond the drape.

"Where's Jeff!" I demand.

A door to the operating room swings open. "Found him," says a nurse, positioning her facemask over her mouth. "He was in the phone booth. Says he'll be here in a minute. He's putting on scrubs."

A sigh of relief escapes my mouth, and I don't feel a thing as one of the obstetric surgeons makes an eight-inch horizontal incision above my pubic bone.

"Wrong door!" someone barks. My husband comes into view with a surgical cap on his head and a mask over his nose and mouth. Even with half his face covered, I can tell he's grimacing as a nurse guides him past my gaping abdomen to a stool behind my head.

"Sorry," says the nurse to one of the doctors. "Didn't know you'd already cut."

"Ewww," Jeff whispers in my ear, adding a bit of levity to a situation that is moving too fast for both of us. Stroking my cheek, he repeats little phrases of encouragement. *You're doing great. This is it. Here we go.* I sense these affirmations are as much for his benefit as mine.

I watch the surgeons from their chests up as they work to extract Clare from my womb. Muffled voices volley brief commands back and forth. I hear words like *distress* and *stat* and *resuscitation.* Then the voices go silent, and above the surgical drape I see one of the doctors holding a limp little body covered in blood and mucus and some other dark goo. She isn't moving. *My baby isn't moving!*

Everything will be fine, everything will be fine, everything will be fine. I repeat these four words to myself as a mantra, a mandate even.

No congratulations are offered. No baby is placed gently in my arms.

More people in surgical scrubs seem to appear from nowhere and surround Clare. Hushed voices cut the whir of activity, as she is moved to another table across the room. Jeff moves back and forth between Clare and me, trying to see what he can at her table, trying not to see what is below the surgical drape at mine. About a dozen people are in the room now, most of them focused on Clare. Their close-knit huddle blocks my view. I strain to see her but cannot, so I turn my head away and squeeze my eyes shut, sending tears into the light blue surgical cap covering my hair.

Everything will be fine, everything will be fine, everything will be fine.

The activity around Clare increases and Jeff comes back to my side. He looks frightened, more than I've ever seen before. And I need him not to be frightened. I need him to be certain and strong. Because I no longer am.

"They said she passed a stool in utero and choked on it. They're about to move her to another part of the hospital," he says. "To the intensive care unit for newborns." Above his surgical mask, Jeff's eyes reflect the terror I'm feeling.

Several people push the incubation cart holding Clare toward the operating room exit. "Stay with the baby, honey," I say to Jeff. "I'll be fine." He gives me a quick kiss, then falls in step with her entourage.

I close my eyes and try convincing myself that Clare will be okay, that bad things happen to other people, not to us. As my self-assurance withers, I switch tactics and begin bargaining with a god I mostly believe in, but sometimes doubt. *Please*, I plead silently, *please, please, please. If something bad is destined for Clare, give it to me instead.* As the surgeons stitch my abdomen shut, I repeat my request, this prayer of the intermittent believer.

Please.

That evening, still groggy from surgery, I smile when Liz pokes her head into my hospital room. "Hey, you," she says, without a trace of her usual acerbic wit. Her husband, Rick, follows behind, holding a duffle bag with the items Jeff requested: toiletries, my bathrobe, jeans and a sweatshirt for Jeff, my date book, our cell phones, the camcorder. He hands the supply bag to my husband and shoots footage of us while we all await the arrival of my baby for a brief visit from the neonatal ICU. Jeff, still wearing his delivery room scrubs, his white surgical mask dangling around his neck, crouches next to me as I lie in the hospital bed waving to the camera and sounding slightly disoriented as I try to explain what happened.

"Well," I say in a slurred voice, "things didn't go quite as I had planned."

Jeff lightly strokes my forearm with his fingers. His tone is one of *c'est la vie* as he recounts the ups and downs of the day and the happy ending we are experiencing now that night has fallen. It's been four hours since Clare's alarming arrival into the world and she's doing surprisingly well. Her Apgar scores have improved. Supplemental oxygen has been discontinued. No apparent health risks remain. And even with her three-and-a-half-weeks-early arrival, she weighs an impressive eight pounds, nine ounces.

I appear to be doing well too, resting in a regular Labor & Delivery room after what seems to have been a textbook case of sudden-onset preeclampsia. "It's as if the mother has an allergic reaction to being pregnant," my obstetrician told us before sending me to the hospital. "And once we deliver your baby, you'll feel better too," she added. Reassurances from various doctors and nurses have been plentiful. *Close call, but everything's okay now. The worst is behind you. It's over.* I believe them all and feel nothing but relief. The story of Clare's dramatic birth will be added to the collection of crazy Lauren and Jeff stories, like how we got engaged on our second date.

There's a soft knock at the door and a nurse enters holding Clare, wrapped snugly in a flannel baby blanket, looking like a giant burrito with a face. A thin cotton cap in muted pastels covers her nearly bald head. Rick and Liz and Jeff all lean in to coo at her, joking about her drama-queen nature and the genetic probability that she gets it from me. When visiting hours end, Jeff thanks our friends for taking care of Spike for the night and walks them to the door. Liz and Rick say their goodbyes and leave us to our privacy as a new family.

The nurse places Clare in my arms, careful not to put any pressure on the area surrounding my stitches. I'm unable to stop staring at her, this little soul who chose me to be her mama. Jeff turns on the camcorder and leans over both of us for a close-up.

"What's the first word that comes to mind?" I hear him ask off to the side.

"Miraculous," I say.

2

SLEEP. I JUST WANT SLEEP, but they keep fussing with me. A nurse tucks my hair into a blue surgical cap. Another swabs my neck with iodine. Jeff is talking and I try to focus on his words, his face. He says something about a central line, that they need to insert one in my neck. *Whatever,* I think. As long as I can sleep. I can barely stay awake even though people are talking to me, at me, and about me. Go away. Let me sleep.

It's four in the morning and I have no memory of all the disruptions during the night: the three times the crash cart slammed into my room, the flashlights shined in my eyes, the fluids hung on my IV pole—the commotion. I have no understanding of what Jeff has already gone through in watching the Blue Team's repeated attempts to stabilize me while I lay unconscious, how surreal his first night as a father has been.

"Even with the topical anesthesia, this is going to hurt a bit," the on-call doctor says, his voice apologetic. "Try not to move." He jabs the right side of my neck and a searing pain slices through my sleepy haze like a laser. I adopt an air of stoicism, an unconvincing attempt at maintaining control.

"Damn," he says. Then he jabs again. And again.

I see Jeff wince every time the needle pierces my skin. It's a look that says he would take my place in a heartbeat if he could. Blood leaks from my neck onto the pillow, and the doctor tells Jeff he's having trouble getting the needle into my jugular in the proper position. Someone lifts my head and places a large pad under it, as I make what I think is a joke about vampires. No one laughs. I'm not entirely sure what is happening, but I can feel each attack on my neck, each attempt by the doctor, whose frustration registers on his face. He asks my husband to step back because this may be too much for him to watch. Jeff complies and a nurse pulls the curtain around my bed, leaving my husband to rely on his imagination as the doctor and I both swear repeatedly—he because he's unable to secure the central line, me because it hurts like hell.

The central line is finally secured and someone pulls back the curtain. Jeff approaches the bed and the doctor explains that I need to go back into surgery as soon as possible because I'm not responding to the "fluid boluses." Jeff says he doesn't understand. I don't either, but I don't care. I just want all these people to leave so I can sleep in peace. The doctor says that my repeated blood pressure drops indicate that I'm hemorrhaging internally and they need to find out why. They've booked the OR. The surgeons are on their way. Please sign these papers.

03/03/00—At 6:30 a.m., Jeff called us to say that Lauren was bleeding internally and that the doctors were going to operate through her original incision to repair it. He broke down on the phone and could hardly talk. Fluid and blood were collecting in her abdomen. Legs, ankles, feet, face, hands—all puffy and distended. I made arrangements to fly out immediately.

I awaken in a hospital bed, my body still numb from the general anesthesia, bags of ice covering my belly. The room is full: Jeff, Mom, girlfriends Liz and Pam, my brother Tim. And Clare. Tim holds my baby, walking around the room and speaking softly to her as he gently bobs up and down. Mom sits in the corner writing in a blue spiral-bound notebook. Someone notices that I have opened my eyes and familiar faces lean in toward me.

"How're you feeling?" I hear. My throat hurts too much to speak, an aftereffect of the breathing tube that pumped oxygen into my lungs during my latest surgery. Instead, I simply nod my head.

With Clare still in his arms, Tim approaches the foot of the bed, a wicked smile playing on his face.

"Hey," he says, "If you die, can I have your bike?"

It's an age-old family joke that elicits a scowl from our mother every time my siblings and I say it to one another, usually when one of us is embarking on a lengthy journey or precarious endeavor. "I love you" has never come easily for my family, humor being the more common expression of affection. The fact that Tim is using the bike joke now tells me everything must be okay.

I drift in and out of consciousness, grasping pieces of conversations about me. I hear my family comparing notes, questioning doctors, and accepting small comforts from the nurses: the extra time taken to explain medical terms, recommendations for a good sandwich shop nearby, general reassurances about my prognosis.

When the latest blood test results arrive, one of the doctors explains that they don't reflect the kind of recovery pattern expected in a preeclampsia patient. Although there is no definitive cure for this pregnancy-related disorder, delivering the baby typically sets the recovery process in motion for the mother, the baby, or both. But I'm proving to be anything but typical. My body isn't producing the clotting factors needed after surgery, and since this morning my platelet count has dropped to 54,000, normal being 150,000 to 450,000. Round-the-clock blood transfusions replenish my vascular system while my own blood continues to leak through my vessels and veins, filling my abdomen, which is now much larger than when I was pregnant. The ongoing blood loss can no longer be blamed on the few small "bleeders" discovered and repaired during the surgery earlier today. It is now attributed to DIC—Disseminated Intra-vascular Coagulation, the failure of the blood to clot. Because of its high fatality rate, medical professionals—behind closed doors—also define DIC as Death Is Certain.

03/04/00—I called Elizabeth [a good friend] *and told her what was going on. She said the first thing she wanted me to do was to not think that Lauren was going to die, that she was going to be okay, but we'd need to work on it. I was to picture Lauren healthy. When I put that picture in my head, what I got was Clare just beginning to walk, tottering along, with Lauren in front of her, mimicking Clare's walk and looking back at Clare and laughing with her.*

"I want a Coke," I say to no one in particular. I just woke up and my voice is deep and gravelly, my throat still raw from yesterday's breathing tube. The room is empty except for a nurse, who laughs at my request. She thinks I'm kidding.

I'm not. I want a Coke. Now.

"Where's Jeff?" I ask.

"I think he went to get coffee," she says.

My nasal passages ache, and when I touch my face I realize there's a hard plastic tube the width of a pencil coming out of my left nostril, leading to a clear container hanging off the side of the bed. Murky gray fluid lines the bottom of the container, maybe half a cup's worth. A pint-sized bag of blood hangs from a tall thin metal pole on the other the side of my bed, a thinner tube running from the bag to my body. My mouth is parched. I haven't had anything to eat or drink since the small cup of water I was given at the doctor's office while trying to produce a urine sample. That was two days ago.

"I'm serious," I whisper. "I really want a Coke."

"I'm sorry, Lauren," says my nurse. "You're not allowed to have food or liquids yet. You have to pass gas before we can get you something to drink."

"I have to *fart* to get a Coke?"

Food and beverages will cause problems if my guts are still asleep, she explains. Once I start passing gas, they'll know the anesthesia has worn off, and it will be safe for me to eat and drink again.

"Besides, it wouldn't stay in your stomach anyway," she says, pointing to the tube in my nose. "That's sucking everything out, including all the fluids your stomach is producing on its own." I glance again at the plastic container attached to the end of my nasal tubing. *Ick.*

"If everything is being sucked out anyway, why can't I have a Coke?" I'm not willing to give up without a fight, and her expression tells me she's considering my argument. I'm making headway. Flashes of the old relentless negotiator in me spring forth to seal the deal.

"Come on," I say. "I'll let you do anything to me that you need to, if you'll give me a Coke first."

"Let's check with the doc when he gets here. If he says it's okay, I promise I'll find you a Coke."

Five, ten minutes later, a doctor enters my room. The nurse explains my request and the doctor pauses as if weighing the pros and cons.

"Sure," he says. "But only a little, 200 cc's at most."

My nurse and I share a smile in joint recognition of our small victory. I have no idea how much 200 cc's is, but I'm thrilled nonetheless. She leaves my room and returns minutes later with a cup of ice and a can of Coke. Pouring some of the soda over the ice and mashing it around with a straw, she tells me she needs to get rid of some of the carbonation just to be on the safe side.

"Small sips," she says, holding the cup to my chin. I put the straw in my mouth and suck, the burning sensation in my throat offset by the wetness in my mouth, the sweet taste on my tongue. And then, *whoosh!* Regurgitated Coke shoots out the tube in my nose, adding a brownish color to the contents already in the container hanging off my bed. The nurse and I laugh at the absurdity of this scene. A few interns and orderlies poke their heads in my room to see what's so funny.

"Watch this!" I croak. I take another sip and once more Coke shoots out my nose. Everyone laughs. More people lean into my room to see what's going on, so I repeat my trick and they respond accordingly. Suddenly the crowd parts and I see Jeff—coffee cup in hand, his face stricken—as he makes his way into the room. He seems confused and out of breath, like he's run down the hallway to get here.

"Hey, honey!" I bark. "Check it out!" I take another sip of Coke and it shoots out my nose. All eyes are on Jeff, awaiting his response.

I promise to keep my sense of humor, my husband had said to me when we exchanged our wedding vows in a redwood forest three years earlier. Then he added, *I know that won't be a problem for you.*

Jeff slowly shakes his head, a smile playing at the corners of his mouth.

03/05/00—Thought for the day: If he were still alive, Lauren's father would have been 64 today. Is he helping her?

The average person has ten to fourteen pints of blood in his body, roughly two pints for every twenty-five pounds of body weight. Now on my fourth day in the hospital, I've been transfused with more than fifty pints. And my body is still not responding the way the doctors had hoped. It's not producing clotting factors, as if I've temporarily become a hemophiliac. My liver shows signs of acute failure. My kidneys are going too. I'm jaundiced, my skin and eyes mustard yellow. A large blood clot is forming on top of my uterus. I must be moved immediately to a hospital that is better equipped to handle my case, one with a surgical intensive care unit and dialysis machinery, which this hospital—primarily a birthing center—does not have.

Jeff sits in the back of the ambulance with me as we drive from San Francisco's Sunset neighborhood to the Fillmore district on a foggy Sunday afternoon. He hasn't been home since his impromptu visit with roses three days ago. My mental capacity diminished, I struggle to work out a simple pun or flippant remark for the ambulance driver, but instead lapse into sadness and confusion. We finish the drive in silence.

At the new hospital, Jeff keeps pace with the paramedics as they push my gurney down hallways, around corners, on and off the elevator, and through the large swinging doors that make a loud *pshhht!* as they automatically open into the surgical ICU. Doctors in white coats stride around with clipboards in hand and interns trailing behind, while nurses duck in and out of patients' rooms, most of which have their sliding doors open and a single family member standing vigil. Someone directs the paramedics to a room in the middle of the unit, right across from the nurses' station. There's a noticeable difference in the atmosphere of this hospital; it's busier, much more high-tech. I groan with pain as I'm transferred from my gurney to a special air mattress.

I'm fading fast and within hours I won't respond to anything except through physical reflexes: the dilation of my pupils in response to a doctor's small flashlight, the jerking of my leg in response to a thumb's firm scrape across the sole of my foot. On a scale of one to ten, with ten being the worst, my team of specialists has deemed me a nine-and-a-half.

03/05/00—Jeff crashed at home around 10:30 p.m. When I went into the master bedroom to give him an update on Lauren, I thought he'd left a night-light on, but it turned out to be candles that were burning on their little altar. When Jeff woke up, he held my hand and said to look at the angel card he'd drawn. It read "Faith."

Preeclampsia is one of the oldest diseases on record, having been first identified and recorded over two thousand years ago. Delivering the baby is the only known treatment, and *usually* the mother improves once the baby is out of her body. But in some cases postpartum complications set in. Preeclampsia can develop into eclampsia and ultimately HELLP Syndrome, both related to preeclampsia and both life-threatening. My own diagnosis has morphed from preeclampsia to HELLP Syndrome to something the doctors can't quite name. So more tests will be run, liver biopsies taken, dialysis administered, and bags of blood transfused.

Each year, preeclampsia claims the lives of roughly 76,000 women worldwide. The number of babies taken by this disorder is even higher: more than half a million. And while most deaths due to preeclampsia and its related complications occur in developing countries, we in the developed world are not immune to its impact. Many of us naïvely believe that women in the West—with all our advancements in medical care—no longer die in childbirth.

But we do.

3

WHEN JEFF AND I SHARED THE NEWS of my pregnancy seven months ago, we made no secret of the fact that it was unplanned. There was, however, one detail we left out: Jeff didn't want to have children.

In the spring of 1999, I had left a job that I was ill suited for, and at my husband's encouragement, I put on a backpack and traveled throughout Europe for six weeks before launching my search for another corporate position as a VP of marketing. Jeff joined me for the first two weeks, but work demands required his return after that. A month later, I flew home to the San Francisco airport wearing a clingy French minidress, Italian pumps, and a Mediterranean tan. Time apart had increased our desire and dampened our judgment, and our usual precautions were tossed aside as quickly as our clothes. Within hours of stepping off the plane, I was pregnant.

Weeks later, we stood together in the bathroom staring at a home pregnancy test, its tiny blue plus sign irrevocably changing our future. My internal response was a mosaic of shock and apprehension and joy. For years, I'd imagined that one day a little girl named Clara, named for the angel in my favorite movie, *It's a Wonderful Life*, would be a part of my life. I'd even shared this thought with Jeff after our first date, and before he asked me to marry him four days later, he'd amended her name to Clare. During long nighttime phone conversations early in our relationship, we'd talked about starting a family one day, had even fantasized about getting pregnant on our honeymoon months before we married. But my corporate career and his entrepreneurial company, dinner parties with friends and travel for work dominated our first years of marriage. Thoughts of children, *our* children, were left behind in the flurry of a busy life together. Conversations about Clare were fewer and fewer, until one day Jeff told me he wasn't so sure about having kids. We had a good thing going, he'd said. Why mess with it? He didn't want to lose what he called our *freedom*, didn't want anything infringing on the life we'd created together. And, equally important, he didn't want to forfeit his dream of one day returning to academia and immersing himself in a full-time PhD program. To him, becoming a father was more about sacrifice than integration, giving up his needs and wants instead of simply expanding what we shared to include one more.

"Okay, so you're pregnant," he said, sounding catatonic, before turning and walking out of the bathroom that day. I sat, head in hands, on the edge of the tub and shed tears of panic, of fear, and then, of anger. We'd discussed this before, the game plan should I become pregnant. We'd agreed that abortion would not be the solution for an unplanned pregnancy. *So if I get pregnant?* I'd asked. *We'd become parents*, he'd replied, without a hint of sarcasm. I'd assumed that Jeff's recently voiced aversion to parenthood was directly tied to the pressure of trying to sell his software company. Once that pressure was gone, once our finances stabilized, I'd reassured myself, surely he'd reconsider his position and I'd be one of those forty-something first-time moms.

Jeff worked hard to put on a show of excitement when we phoned our respective families to share the news or when we ran into acquaintances and confirmed the rumors. But at home, just the two of us, he withdrew. His mood was somber, his conversations numb. At night when we read on the couch together, I'd look up from my book to find him staring, expressionless, out the window or at a corner of the ceiling.

Initially, I tried to help him work through his fears. I reminded him of how much we'd both enjoyed that precocious little girl, Mathilde, the daughter of new friends we'd met in France, and how we'd jokingly said that if we could get one like her we'd do it in a heartbeat. I rented Steve Martin's *Parenthood* one night in hopes of showing the comedic side of our situation, but watching the movie made him more anxious. When a friend of mine sent us a book for expectant dads that showed a pinstripe shirt on the cover, Jeff flipped to the table of contents and, shaking his head, read aloud one of the chapter titles: "Money, Money, Money." The book, unread, went in the trash.

I sensed that Jeff sincerely wanted to embrace his impending role as a father, but I also sensed he was lost, clueless as to how to do it. I suggested therapy, a path he'd never taken, and immediately I felt the gates to his receptivity slam shut. Long ago, we'd promised one another that divorce would never be an option for resolving any marital issues we might encounter, but eventually, I'd had enough of trying to console him. I was pissed, surprised at the potency of maternal protectiveness that sprang forth, righteousness for the embryo growing within me. I offered to absolve him of his wedding vows, to let him go so he could pursue the life he'd imagined—without this baby and, consequently, without me. Jeff's expression told me I'd never say more hurtful words to him.

"Don't you know I'd never leave you?" he said, his eyes tearing up.

I know that, I thought. *But I won't allow this baby to grow up in a household of stifled resentment. If need be, I'll leave you.*

What would it be like to raise a child alone? Would I be able to provide for her and still spend time with her? Would she ask about her father? When I was two months pregnant, these were the questions I turned over in my mind. Not questions about diaper services or breast pumps, but about my marriage. I discussed my fears with no one, not even Jeff. I felt I'd already lost him. Now it was a matter of choosing to stay with this new resigned Jeff, the one whose *joie de vivre* had seemingly been extinguished, or to move on.

Then one day, it happened. A crack. Small, barely noticeable, but a crack nonetheless.

"Could you give me the number of that shrink you mentioned?" Jeff asked nonchalantly, as he cleared the table after dinner. I squelched my elation, afraid of overreacting.

"Sure," I said, my composure matching his.

A week later, Jeff returned from his first therapy session. "So how was it?" I asked, again careful not to come across as being too eager.

"It was okay, I guess," he said. "She sure doesn't say much." I let it drop.

The following week, Jeff returned from his second session.

"Honey, I am so fucked up!" he said, laughing. "Not only do I have a fear of failure, but I also have a fear of success. You'd think I could just average the two together and be normal." As Jeff shared his insights from therapy, it was obvious he'd turned a corner and, though still anxious about parenthood, was making progress.

Two weeks later, I was visiting Mom and my stepdad, John, in Boulder, when Jeff called the day after his fourth appointment, exuberant. At the therapist's prompting, he'd taken a close look at what exactly he stood to lose by becoming a father. He realized it wasn't our freedom. It wasn't our romance. It wasn't our ability to travel or get together with friends. What he couldn't get past, he told me, was his self-imposed idea that fatherhood meant working a steady, and likely soul-crushing, job until retirement. Worse yet, it meant relinquishing his desire to return to school. PhD programs took time: six to eight years, and money: tens of thousands in tuition and books, not to mention the loss of income for the duration of the program. He told me how he couldn't sleep last night, agitated by thoughts of losing his academic dream, so he got out of bed and did something he'd never done his entire adult life. He made a personal budget, calculating how much money he'd need for graduate school, as well as for major family expenses such as a down payment on a home, our child's college education, and other expenses that grown-ups concern themselves with. And that, he explained, is when the breakthrough occurred.

If Jeff could sell his software company, which was struggling financially, he might walk away with enough money to earmark some of it for school. And even if the company went under, he realized he could earn money another way and then focus on his academic goals. Viewing our situation with this newfound clarity, he told me, led to an even more remarkable occurrence. He regained his sense of hope.

My best friend, my partner in life, had returned to me.

Less than a month later, as if by some cosmic reward system, Jeff came home late one night with a big grin on his face and an even bigger check in his hand. He and his business partners, along with a gaggle of attorneys, had worked until nearly midnight finalizing the sale of the company. Giddy, we sat side by side on the couch for over an hour staring at his portion of the proceeds, a percentage of which would be deposited into two college funds. One for Clare. And one for Jeff.

4

NEITHER JEFF NOR CLARE IS WORTH the excruciating physical pain I feel. This is what I tell my husband during one of my brief periods of consciousness after he begs me to do what the doctors have said is crucial: to get mad and start fighting. I spew hurtful statements without concern for Jeff's feelings, for what he has endured on very little sleep for five days. Hepatic encephalopathy is causing the neurons in my brain to misfire, the liver specialist tells Jeff, and that's fueling my desire to lash out. Every change in my position made by well-intentioned nurses sends a white-hot searing jolt through my midsection. Liver and kidney failure conspire with gallons of hemorrhaged blood trapped in my abdomen, wracking my body with an indescribable agony, the steady flow of morphine seemingly no help at all. My deep guttural groans and intermittent screams are heard throughout the ICU and with enough frequency that some of the younger staff, I will later learn, secretly nickname me The Screamer.

My only focus right now is the pain—or more accurately, ending it. If that means slipping away without a fight, so be it.

"Just let me go," I say to Jeff.

Preeclampsia is a systemic disease. It attacks the liver, kidneys, vascular system, and lungs. Clearly, with all the blood transfusions I've received so far, my vascular system is in failure. The latest lab results show that my liver and kidneys have lost more ground. Now my doctors want to gauge my mental acuity, so they discontinue the use of the intravenous pain medication. My level of confusion and unresponsiveness increases and is no longer attributed to the morphine. This is not good news. It's a sign that I'm quickly moving toward the final stage of liver failure, perhaps a coma.

03/06/00—Lauren seems to be slipping away in spite of everyone's best efforts.

Tim's wife, Dede, arrives from Orange County and enters my ICU room as I launch into a fit, no longer under the calming spell of morphine. With both hands, I blindly thrash at the hard plastic tube in my left nostril, the same one that shot soda out of my stomach yesterday morning. The nurse assigned to care for me is in the next room with her other patient, the ICU having a two-to-one patient-to-nurse ratio. Jeff grabs at my forearms to prevent me from hurting myself.

"Get help!" he yells. Dede leaves without a word and soon one of the medical residents rushes in. He secures my arms to the bars on either side of my bed with Velcro-and-canvas restraints, careful not to tangle them with my IV line, transfusion line, or any of the other myriad tubes running from my arms, chest, and head to various medical devices. I succumb to the restraints and Jeff releases his grip. He walks around the bed and gives Dede a hug as she dissolves into tears.

Discussions about my prognosis no longer include me. My personal support team—Jeff, my mom and stepdad, Tim, my sisters Karen and Steph, brother-in-law Mark, Liz, Pam, and another close friend, Sabra—regularly meets with the medical specialists to discuss my care. These "summit meetings," as they will come to be called by my family, take place in the ICU waiting room, sometimes twice a day. A liver transplant is discussed, but for now the doctors want to take a wait-and-see approach.

My current treatment plan involves lab work every few hours and continuous blood transfusions until my body gives some clear indication of next steps. Called "supportive care," this is what doctors often do when they enter unknown territory, when—as the liver specialist puts it—the *science* of medicine becomes the *art* of medicine.

03/07/00—I went to the hospital tonight and went into Lauren's ICU cubicle by myself, when no one else was with her. She was completely unresponsive. Her lips were curled back from her teeth and her eyes looked like those of a newborn baby bird—big and kind of sunken. She was completely unresponsive to my touch. I whispered in her ear what Elizabeth had said about Capricorns being able to overcome the biggest obstacles, and that she had the ability to get well again. No response.

I went back to the waiting room and, crying, told John that I had to go home, that I couldn't handle seeing Lauren as she was. As we waited for the elevator to come, Tim and Jeff came over and held me as they reassured me that Lauren was going to get well. I let them talk and tried to listen, but the whole time I thought, They're fools if they think that body in that condition will get better. They're just deluding themselves.

Several pieces of my liver are removed through an opening in my neck, and I don't feel a thing. I'm semicomatose, and the morphine drip that was temporarily discontinued yesterday has been reinstated. Normally, liver biopsies are performed through the belly, but my midsection is now the size of a medium Fitball. I weigh two hundred and sixty pounds—sixty pounds over my highest pregnancy weight and a hundred pounds over my normal weight.

The biopsy reports come back. No microvesicular fatty cells, so fatty-liver pregnancy is ruled out. No cirrhosis, so too much partying in college is ruled out. No hepatitis A, B, or C, and no sign of chronic disease. Yet the latest round of blood work shows that my coagulation numbers have gotten worse since the last set of lab tests was done four hours ago. I'm now a Status One on the liver transplant list. I have, in effect, cut to the front of a very long line because of my age, favorable health history, lack of previous medical challenges, and the urgency of my situation.

Each year, tens of thousands of people wait on organ transplant lists. They wait for someone else to die in a manner conducive to saving and recycling the major organs, eyes, and usable tissues of the body. They wait for the loved ones of the recently departed to acknowledge and respect the existence of an organ donation card, to see beyond their grief and offer up parts of the deceased body that can save the lives of others. And each year, in this country alone, more than 6,000 people die waiting.

The next morning's lab results indicate that I had a good night. I also had two bowel movements while I slept, a sign that the ammonia by-products linked to the toxicity in my body are now exiting my system. *She's going to make it,* declares my team of specialists. I've dropped three pounds, down to two hundred and fifty-seven. Good news indeed. By mid-morning my fluid output exceeds my fluid input by 200 cc's an hour. More good news. And by early afternoon, the doctors have discontinued the blood transfusions, including the FFP—fresh frozen plasma—that they've been weaning me off since last night. (Months from now I will hear the story of how slaphappy Tim, Karen, Steph, Mark, and Sabra were in the family waiting room after reviewing what they'd just learned in the daily summit meeting. They couldn't remember what the acronym FFP stood for, so they pondered names like Freeze-dried Frozen Plasma and Fresh Fucking Plasma. But knowing that plasma is only one component of whole blood, they decided to forget the acronym and go with the term Blood Light.)

The good news is short-lived. Within twenty-four hours the Blood Light transfusions resume. As more blood bags are on their way from the local blood center, my baby is on her way to the airport with Tim and Dede, who will act as her guardians indefinitely. I'm aware of neither of these details.

03/08/00—Blood Centers of the Pacific notified the hospital that its supplies are rapidly being depleted. I decided that it would be better if I just stayed at Lauren's home, managing the house, handling all the phone calls, and requesting that people give blood instead of sending flowers.

Somewhere, a hospital monitor goes off. *Beep! Beep! Beep!*

"Honey!" Jeff yells, his voice filled with panic. I open my eyes for the first time in days and look at my husband.

"I thought you'd stopped breathing," he says.

A nurse rushes into my room. "That alarm was in the next room," she says.

Eyelids drooping, I smile at Jeff, a crooked smile—he later tells me—that says *Silly man. I need my rest and I'm going back to sleep now.* Without saying a word, I close my eyes and return to the place I have been on and off since Clare's birth almost a week ago, a place I will have trouble describing to others later, let alone remembering clearly. Red rock canyons like the ones in Sedona, Arizona, that I hiked years ago with Spike. Warmth. Lots of warmth and light. The feeling that I am bundled snugly, the same way my baby is in the photographs that hang on the wall—a subtle plea to those caring for me that this patient is a mother now, in need of their utmost attention. In this surreal place I go I have the sense that my body is healing, that I am being nurtured and protected. By whom or by what I don't know. But I like it here. And I want to stay.

5

I CAN ONLY EXPLAIN what happened two weeks before Clare's birth as the freakiest of coincidences, or angels in action.

It was late afternoon on a weekday and I was strolling along the water's edge at Fort Funston beach with an old friend who was in town on business. As Spike darted in and out of the rising tide, Dean and I talked about our thoughts on becoming parents: his through a recent adoption, and mine as a mother-to-be. We shared our fears about having children, our dreams for their future, and we teased one another about how much we'd matured since those carefree days as graduate school roommates, when our greatest concerns centered around midterms, summer internships, and our respective love lives.

Leaving the beach, we returned to my SUV, and I pulled out of the parking lot heading south on Highway 1 so we could make a U-turn a quarter-mile down the road that would redirect us north toward my home. I had pulled onto that highway at that exact location dozens of times before, as Spike and I were frequent visitors to Fort Funston. The drivers on this stretch of winding two-lane road are generally aware and respectful of cars pulling out of the parking lot and merging with traffic. But this time, the driver on my left would not let me merge to get into the U-turn lane. When I went faster to pull in front of him, he went faster. When I slowed down to pull in behind him, he slowed down. No matter what I did, he stayed with me. I reduced my speed to a near stop and pulled into the U-turn lane, making a mental note about how strange his driving was. Not infuriating—his antics delayed us by mere seconds—just odd. We made our U-turn and headed north.

Minutes later, a metal-on-metal crashing noise interrupted our conversation, and I looked at the oncoming lane to see a late-model sedan rebound off the back of a camper van and careen across the road, coming straight toward us at an alarming speed. Like a bullet, the car shot in front of our path, up the curb, and across a popular jogging trail before dropping out of sight in the direction of the lake less than fifty yards off the road. Instinctively, I pulled over and kicked into crisis-management mode. My protruding belly precluded me from traversing the heavy brush covering the hillside, so Dean ran down to the lake without me. I dialed 911 on my cell phone while simultaneously stopping a bicyclist and directing him down the hill to help the rescue effort. Another witness to the accident pulled over and asked me to watch his two-year-old daughter so he could go down to the lake, too.

I watched from atop the hill as Dean and the other two men stood chest-deep in the water, struggling to open the car doors, pounding on the windows, shouting, whatever they could to get the driver to respond. And then the car slipped below the lake's surface.

Fire trucks, an ambulance, police cars, and television news crews arrived, one in a helicopter overhead. The rush-hour traffic backed up as far as I could see. A team of medical emergency divers emerged from the lake carrying the limp body of an elderly woman. They laid her on the grass about ten feet from the road and I noticed that her left shoe was missing. EMTs surrounded her, cutting off her dress in full view of the twenty or so pedestrians who had gathered. More than thirty minutes had passed since her car plunged into the lake, yet the medics worked on her at least that long trying to restore her pulse. Dean stood off to the side, trembling, his shoulders draped in a thin blanket given to him by a passerby. He was chilled, his clothing sodden, and he seemed to be experiencing a mild level of shock. I called Jeff and told him we'd be late, and in the middle of explaining what had happened, my cell phone battery died. The EMTs loaded the woman into the back of an ambulance and drove her to the hospital, where she would be pronounced DOA—dead on arrival.

The sun had long since set before the accident investigators were able to question Dean and me about what we'd seen. I asked them almost as many questions as they asked me, learning that the driver had likely had a heart attack that caused her to lose consciousness, the dead weight of her foot accelerating her car into the camper van before rebounding toward the lake. She may have been dead before her car even reached the lake, the investigator said. Or maybe she drowned.

As Dean and I drove back to my house, the mood in the car was somber. I reassured him that he'd done everything he could, but he just stared out the window into the evening drizzle.

At home, Jeff was waiting, anxious. All he knew was that I'd almost been the victim of a head-on collision. I had no idea that his response to my close call would be so disproportionate to the situation. With more than a month until my due date, he suggested that I shouldn't drive anywhere until after Clare was born. I flatly refused, arguing that he was being irrational and that if viewed another way, perhaps the otherwise tragic event was a sign, a *good* sign. How else could I explain the brief delay caused by the driver who wouldn't allow me to merge into his lane? Narrowly escaping an accident that would've surely been fatal for me felt like a message.

"It's not my time," I told Jeff repeatedly. "Don't you see? It's not my time."

For days, he continued to implore me not to drive, and each time I launched into my "it's not my time" speech, sometimes patiently, other times not.

Three weeks later, with my life teetering in a delicate balance, I wonder if my words ever danced at the edge of his consciousness, imploring him to have faith, to hold fast to the knowledge that eventually I'd come back to him.

It's not my time.

6

KAREN HOLDS TINY MOIST SPONGES on sticks to my mouth and I snap at them like a turtle, my neck straining against gravity. My lips are chapped, my throat parched. Wild with thirst, I refuse to release the occasional stick I manage to clamp down on with my teeth. Worried that I'll inadvertently choke myself on a sponge, Karen switches to a moist washcloth, holding it to my mouth and allowing me to suck small amounts of water from it. She speaks softly, lovingly, imploring me to release the washcloth, coaxing me with promises of more moisture if I comply. Only small amounts of liquid are permitted, and this approach is the safest way to ensure that I won't gulp too much water at once.

"Ouch!" yells Karen when she momentarily looks away and I bite her fingers. It is not the gentle nibble of a teasing younger sister but a full-fledged bite, that of a crazed animal caught in a leg trap. She seems annoyed, but quickly regains her composure. Her work with institutionalized elderly patients has been good training for dealing with a little sister who has been reduced to the most basic level of functioning. Right now that translates to trying to satisfy an almost unbearable thirst.

The nurse assigned to my case for the day enters my room. Noticing the smell of another bowel movement, she tells Karen they'll need to change my bedsheets and clean my behind. Karen leans in close and whispers in my ear.

"Lauren, we have to clean you up," she says. "They have to roll you on your side again."

I groan and speak my first words in three days. "Oh god."

"No, Wa," Karen says, calling me by the nickname her daughter gave me when she was just a toddler. "I think you mean, 'Oh dog.'" Karen's remarks are a nod to the old joke, a favorite of our family's, about the dyslexic agnostic insomniac who stays up all night wondering if there's a dog. But in my weakened mental state, I have no idea what she's talking about. *What dog?*

Another nurse, with a ponytail and mannerisms that are far too perky for my liking, pokes her head into my room. "I'll help you roll yours if you help me roll mine," she says to my nurse. Her voice is nauseatingly chipper and she makes no attempt to acknowledge my presence, despite the fact that *I* am that which is about to be rolled. Karen steps to the side, allowing the two women to deal with my latest mess.

"Are you ready, Lauren?" my nurse asks. Without waiting for my answer, she and her rolling partner begin heaving my inert body onto its right side, like a couple of marine biologists trying to maneuver a beached manatee back to the safety of the ocean after a violent storm. I try to protest, but the words are caught in my throat, trumped by an excruciating pain in my abdomen. Multiple organ failure and movement are not a good combination, no matter how much morphine is being pumped through one's veins.

I feel the scurry of activity that's taking place behind my back: the practiced and efficient movements of the nurses' hands wiping my bottom, the balling up of the soiled sheet, and the snapping of a fresh clean sheet in its place. All the while I'm quietly counting to ten, as my nurse instructed me to do when my moaning began. Does reaching ten mean she'll roll me carefully back the way I was? I don't know, but for now I have a focus, a goal: just make it to ten.

I reach the number eight and find myself being carefully lowered to my back. I'm remarkably grateful for the small reprieve offered by those last two unspoken digits. As my body begins to regain its equilibrium, the nurse again asks me to count to ten, and the thought of what comes next overwhelms me. *Not again. Not again. Please-please-please not again.* But again, I am hoisted onto my side, this time to the left. One final tug of the fresh sheet and I'm lowered onto my back, having counted only to three.

"There you go, Lauren," says my nurse. "I'll bet that feels better without all that poop, huh?"

I disagree, but say nothing. She wouldn't understand. None of them would. The truth is, I enjoy shitting myself. It's warm, comforting, and I prefer lying in my feces to the painful acrobatics that accompany the cleanup process. Lately, nothing seems to be in my control and all too often, people speak about me as if I'm not there or I'm a helpless, dependent baby. Keeping my bowel movements a secret is my way of exerting control in a world where I've been stripped of my independence.

03/10/00—At 9:30 a.m., Lauren opened her eyes, looked around the room, then at Karen, and asked, "Where the fuck am I? What day is this? Where is everybody?" She's back!

I open my eyes and scan the room, struggling to understand the scenario before me, like awakening after a deep sleep and momentarily struggling to place oneself in time and circumstance. The only other person in the room is my sister Karen, and we live on opposite sides of the country. *What's she doing here?* I have no recollection of our spending the past two days together. Karen moves closer to my bed, leans in, and smiles.

"Well, hello, Princess," she says, using the same voice she used to use when her kids were toddlers. Then her tone changes to mock anger.

"Boy, do you owe me big-time," she says. I do not know that during one of my family's black-humor moments in the waiting room they made jokes about how I couldn't die, as that would deprive them of the pleasure of killing me for putting them through this emotional nightmare. I scan my memory for clues as to why I owe her. I remember something about a baby shower. And a baby. I look more closely around the room, searching to find baby gifts that Karen may have given me, perhaps one that warrants owing her "big-time," such as the purple extra-tall baby jogger I listed on a registry once, though I'm not sure when. But there are no baby joggers, no baby gifts, no babies. I have no sense that I'm lying in a hospital bed, that I'm gravely ill. What I do have is that sense of being on the outside looking in, of joining a group of laughing people and not being in on the joke. I'm embarrassed by my lack of understanding, so I say nothing.

But then it makes sense. It's this place, this hideous mauve-walled "house" with the torn curtain hanging from the sliding glass doors that separate this "bedroom" from what I believe is the kitchen. Karen has bought this home in Colorado for me, a home that Jeff and I always said we'd get someday when we were ready to leave San Francisco. And look at that, outside the window: an amazing view of the Rockies! (In reality, the mountains I see are several tall buildings on the north side of San Francisco.) This is a more extravagant gift than I could have imagined, but this place needs serious work. It's butt ugly. I don't want to hurt Karen's feelings, so I won't redecorate until she leaves town. And the minute she does, I'll start by replacing those god-awful striped curtains, the ones with the gaping tear near the top.

How could she possibly afford this gift? It must be all those people, those strangers hovering in the kitchen about fifteen feet away. They are my roommates, I decide, boarders whose rental payments will cover the mortgage. Most of them obviously work from home, *my* home, as technicians of some sort, what with the white lab coats they wear. They're crowded around an erasable white board on the wall, right next to the "cheese cave" (an office off the nurses' station), and making changes to the board with a black marker. That board must be our meal-planning system. After all, with so many people living here we must plan our meals efficiently.

Augh! There's that roommate I loathe, the twenty-something Middle Eastern guy with a black goatee and intense eyes. I can't remember his name or why I despise him so. I have no idea that his name is Michael, or that he's a third-year medical resident, or that he has spent many long nights working to save my life. I hate that man, and I want him out of my home—mortgage payment or no mortgage payment.

I share none of these thoughts with my sister, with anyone.

03/10/00——Karen mentioned to Lauren how beautiful Clare is and how well she's doing, and Lauren seemed sad. Karen wasn't sure if it was because Lauren didn't know if or when she was getting out of the hospital, so Karen decided not to say any more about Clare unless Lauren asks.

My sanity fluctuates like the tides: one minute within view, hours later nowhere in sight. During morning rounds, I'm lucid enough to remember that I'm in a hospital, that something has gone terribly wrong with my health. The doctors are at the door to my room, ready to discuss my case in front of me, but not with me. They ask my sister to leave the room.

"Lauren, the doctors are here and they need to see you," Karen says.

"Just tell them I'm fine!" I say, loud enough for them to hear. I laugh at my own joke.

Karen leaves the room, but returns once the doctors have moved on. She finds a jar of antifungal powder on my bedside table and conducts her own examination of my ravaged body.

Pulling back the thin blanket covering my belly, she peers at my crotch, which I myself cannot see over my inflated belly. Her expression tells me it's a mess down there. She applies some of the powder while simultaneously scrunching up her face in mock disgust for my entertainment. Then she gently maneuvers a folded blanket under my butt to elevate and air out the irritated area. Being with Karen makes me feel safe, like when we were kids and Vance Lanardi tried to trip me at the ice-skating pond. She went after him like a lion after prey, and I never had to worry about Vance bullying me again.

It's lunchtime and I'm about to make my first attempt at eating food that's not ingested through a tube in my nose. With many other patients needing to be hand-fed, my nurse asks Karen to feed me. We start with a box of Resource, a nutrient-rich medicinal beverage that has no business being called a beverage. Even delusional, I can tell this stuff tastes like liquefied chalk. Karen holds the straw to my lips.

"C'mon, Wa, you know you really love this stuff," she says. Her playful teasing works wonders and she gets an entire eight-ounce carton down my throat.

"Good girl," she says. "Now let's see how you do with some real food."

At my sister's request, the hospital cafeteria prepared a meal that's familiar to me. Karen takes the saucer from under the unused coffee mug and scoops a kid-sized portion of tuna salad from the entrée onto the smaller, less intimidating plate. She instinctively understands that as a critically ill patient, I have become almost childlike in my emotional capacity, best fed as one would feed a toddler.

"Small bites," she says, holding a teaspoon of food to my mouth. "Don't overdo it. That-a-girl."

When I finish eating my tuna, Karen offers me sherbet. Again, small bites. Slow and steady. Everything about Karen's approach is spot-on. Her voice, her words, her presence all make me feel safe, even proud of myself for the simple act of eating. Anyone observing this scene wouldn't see a trace of the love-hate relationship we shared well into our twenties. Just a big sister helping her little sister in the most loving way possible—simply being there for her, helping with the basics.

For most of the afternoon, I continue to chatter, sometimes making sense, mostly not.

"I can't believe I had two babies!" I exclaim.

And later: "Jeff, we really need to have another baby as soon as possible!"

Still later: "Tim and Dede are buying us a new house, hon!"

"That's wonderful," Jeff replies. His voice is flat, sounding almost catatonic.

My father-in-law arrives from Michigan late in the afternoon. "Rud!" I say, as he walks into my room, joining Jeff at my bedside. "If I knew you were coming, I'd've baked a cat!" Everyone laughs in that nervous way people do when an inappropriate joke is told at an elegant cocktail party.

Knowing how much I love Italian cuisine, Sabra brings homemade lasagna to the ICU, and at dinnertime Karen heats a small portion in the hospital cafeteria's microwave. When she puts a spoonful in my mouth, I immediately spit it back at her.

"This is shit food!" I bark. I refuse to eat another bite.

Karen asks me what I'd like to eat instead and I tell her waffles. She tries reasoning with me, telling me that it'll be difficult to find waffles at this time of day. When I insist, my father-in-law offers to venture into the neighborhood to find an open waffle house. He returns over an hour later, exhausted from his walk through the city, and proudly opens the to-go box in his hands. I peer inside and see two large golden brown waffles with butter and syrup.

"Waffles!" I snort with disgust. "I'm not eating *those!*"

03/10/00—We all began calling Lauren "the 90% Wa" because she obviously isn't firing on all cylinders. By evening, she seemed so much

better that we were high-fiving and literally dancing in the hall-
way outside the waiting room at the hospital. The relief we felt was
palpable, although I was concerned about Lauren being out of touch
with reality. She had everyone laughing hysterically, but what she
was saying wasn't really her. She was kind of semi-crazy with her
so-called cleverness.

As the evening winds down, so too do my verbal antics. My
vital signs are all stable, as are my latest blood test results. The
central line port going into my jugular vein is capped and additional transfusions are currently on hold. My creatinine levels, the most common indicator of renal function, are back to
normal. The feeding tube I inadvertently ripped from my nasal
passage while sleeping last night will not have to be replaced,
given my recent accomplishment of taking food orally. Things
are looking up, so Jeff agrees to sleep at home tonight for only
the third time in nine days.

"I love you," he whispers in my ear as he gingerly hugs me
goodbye.

"I love you, too," I say. This is the first verbal affection I've
offered Jeff since being transferred to this hospital, since telling
him he wasn't worth all the pain.

"That's what I needed to hear," he replies.

Liz settles into the chair by the window. For the past week,
she, Pam, Sabra, and my family members have made sure that at
least one of them is with me at all times, day and night. Liz has
several more hours until Pam arrives for the midnight-to-five
shift. I try conversing with her, but she repeatedly shushes me.
She moves her chair behind my line of vision, and eventually I
forget she's there and drift off to sleep. All is calm.

I have no memory of Liz leaving for five minutes to get a
latte from the hospital lobby. No memory of my body jerking violently. Of my nurse yelling for help. Of Liz, blocked at
the doorway by someone else. No memory of people in scrubs

holding me down while my body involuntarily fights against their attempts to restrain me. Of the doctor shoving a thick breathing tube down my throat. Of the call Liz made once I was sedated: *Sorry to wake you, Jeff. But you need to get here fast. Lauren just had a grand mal seizure.*

I have no memory of the CT scan that was done to determine if I had a stroke or suffered any brain damage. No memory of lying comatose, hooked up to a breathing machine. Or hours later, conscious again, in arm restraints, gagging, then vomiting from the intrusion of the breathing tube, tears running down my face while I give Jeff a desperate look that says, Why are you letting them do this to me? Why are *you* doing this to me?

7

I DIDN'T PLAN ON GETTING ENGAGED the day after breaking up with someone else. Didn't plan on promising to spend the rest of my life with someone the fourth time I'd ever seen him. I'm a Capricorn. We move slowly, methodically. We do not get engaged willy-nilly—and certainly not on the second date.

To say that when I first met Jeff I "just knew" would be a cliché. To deny it would be a lie. The circumstances under which we met were less than ideal: He had threatened to sue the company I'd recently joined. Less than one month on the job, I was copied on an eight-page letter addressed to the group chairman, which outlined numerous ways we had breached our contract. Despite the professional, even thoughtful, tone of Jeff's letter, I needed to believe he was the enemy. I didn't want to think I'd burned a bridge with my former employer and relocated from one coast to the other only to join a slipshod operation. He *had* to be the bad guy.

On the day of our first meeting, I walked into a conference room extending my arm toward the unfamiliar man who rose to greet me. "Lauren Ward," I said, all business. Jeff shook my hand and simultaneously cupped it with his free hand in what felt like a subtle gesture of intimacy. My three-inch pumps put me at six-feet-four, yet we stood eye to eye. When he introduced himself, I took note of his smooth late-night-radio voice, his deep-set eyes, and strong brow. He looked like an honest man. Late thirties, early forties max. He did not look like a man who would sue one of the world's largest publishers. It was unheard of for our smaller business partners to threaten us with a lawsuit. Not unless they wanted to kiss all future business with every division of our corporate conglomerate goodbye. I couldn't tell if this man put his principles above profit or if he was just plain naïve.

Jeff returned to his seat, and I took an open chair at the opposite end of the table. In the remaining chairs sat one of his business partners and seven of my publishing colleagues. The mood was tense as my boss, Susan, explained that this meeting was about putting past miscommunications behind us. One by one, joint projects between our respective companies were discussed and the tension in the room began to dissipate. I feigned interest, but it was all I could do to maintain a minimal level of focus. Instead, I stared at my notepad and thought about the words that flew through my mind when I'd walked into the room and first set eyes on Jeff as he stood to greet me. *Oh. It's you. What took you so long?*

My boss asked me a question. "Excuse me?" I said, my expression blank. Someone made a joke about my lack of attention and I felt my face burn as everyone laughed. Someone else pointed out that I was blushing, causing more laughter. My eyes swept the room and I saw that Jeff was looking directly at me, smiling, but not laughing. I quickly looked away. Susan repeated the question and I stammered a response that was only remotely relevant. I was certain my colleagues were exchanging glances of doubt about me, the so-called marketing powerhouse they had recruited from a major competitor.

An hour passed and the meeting was adjourned. I made a hasty exit, citing a fictitious conference call. Once inside my office I closed the door and shut the blinds on the floor-to-ceiling windows facing the corridor. Sitting at my desk, I stared out the window at the beautiful wooded area that bordered the building. *What the hell just happened?* I wondered. Why the flustered response to meeting him, and why all those feelings like I've known him before?

Oh. It's you. What took you so long?

Over the next several weeks an abundance of e-mail flew back and forth between our two companies, most of which I was copied on, most of which I ignored or deleted or both. I resolved to discreetly remove myself from any projects involving Jeff's company. My direct involvement was unnecessary, I reasoned. And damn it, I'd just joined this company and wanted to prove that it had been a good decision to hire me. I'd never become personally involved with a professional contact, let alone one who had threatened to sue my company, and I wasn't about to start now. I would not put myself in a position to be gossiped about. Besides, I reminded myself, I'm already dating someone.

Who said anything about dating? my inner voice asked.

One morning there was an e-mail from Jeff in my in-box and I was the only recipient. *Susan suggested that you could help me better understand the intricacies of the college textbook market. Are you free for lunch anytime next week?* There was nothing flirtatious or suggestive about the message, yet alone in my office I once again felt the blood rush to my face. I had spent twelve years in the business world and gone toe-to-toe with some formidable competitors, so why did this particular man make me feel so off balance?

As I reread the e-mail, I worried that agreeing to meet him for lunch would set in motion a domino effect that I was not willing to face. My career was too important and my tenure with the company too brief to risk any rumormongering. I decided I would not have lunch with him. If he wanted to know more about our business, my assistant could set up a group meeting right here at the office.

I was curious, though, in a way that felt like tempting fate. *I'd be happy to meet you for lunch,* I replied. *I'm free on Tuesday.*

I rehearsed my line several times: *"I'm afraid I can't see you— romantically, that is—at least for a year."*

That's what I planned to tell Jeff on our first date, the date I instinctively knew he'd ask me on after our business lunch during which no business was discussed, knew it the minute he asked me if I'd ever been married. No, I'd told him. Just haven't—or did I say *hadn't?*—found the right person. Exact same story, he'd replied.

By the time I returned to work after that lunch, there was already an e-mail from him waiting in my in-box. *I enjoyed myself a great deal and was quite enchanted. If all goes the way I hope it will, we will meet again soon.*

The next day, another e-mail showed up. *I would very much enjoy having dinner with you and taking you out to see this fantastic eighteen-piece big band in North Beach. One of my business partners, Chris, has been leading the Contemporary Jazz Orchestra every Monday night for over a year.*

Monday night sounds fabulous, I replied. Then I wondered how the hell I would sneak out on a date without my boyfriend noticing. Tough to be secretive with the person who is living with you. To be fair, he was staying with me for only a month or so while his new home was being remodeled. But still. I'd never been the cheating kind.

Fate seemed to be sending me a clear message when my boyfriend announced that the renovation was complete and he'd be moving out. Apologizing, he told me he'd be busy settling into his new home and probably wouldn't have much time for me in the coming week. No problem, I said, trying not to inadvertently smile at my good fortune. I helped him pack and kissed him goodbye, feeling less guilty than I should have.

In two nights I would go on a date with Jeff Larsen. And while it felt like I was riding the wave of destiny that delivered this man, quite literally, to my doorstep, I also found myself having to quiet my inner critic, the one that for most of my adult life had implored me to be sensible, to make choices that would be approved of by people who really had no business judging my choices. I wrote my way through conflicting feelings, my head telling me not to be foolish, my heart screaming *Go for it!* Immediately after writing pages in support of keeping my relationship with Jeff platonic for the sake of my career, an opposing vision slipped into my consciousness. *I just had this thought that Chris's band—the jazz orchestra—would be the music at our wedding,* I wrote furiously in my journal. *Weird, but that just popped into my mind.* Then the sober voice of reason retorted *Slow, Lauren, slow.*

Monday night arrived and so did Jeff. I had asked him to meet me at Liz's apartment in the city since I would be spending the night there to avoid a long commute back to the suburbs. It was almost a game for Liz and me, the old meet-me-at-my-friend's-home routine. It was our way of allowing her to check out my suitor du jour. Levelheaded and direct, she was a pretty tough critic, once even shaking her head *no* behind the back of my blind date after less than twenty words were exchanged. (She was right.) But ten minutes after Jeff rang Liz's doorbell, I was surprised—shocked, really—to emerge fully primped from her bathroom and find the two of them laughing and sipping wine in her living room.

One hour and several approving looks from Liz later, Jeff and I left for Jazz at Pearl's nightclub. Between music sets, Jeff's friend Chris visited our table, his conciliatory tone making the animosity between our two companies feel like a thing of the distant past. Jeff and I shared fried calamari and a bottle of chardonnay. I allowed myself to enjoy the evening, decided early on to ditch the speech about our need to be realistic, to keep our relationship as friends only.

Leaving the club, we noticed a considerable drop in the temperature. Jeff took off his coat and wrapped me in it, then drove us back to Liz's apartment, parked the car, and walked me to the door. We stood face-to-face in the bone-chilling summer fog and talked for three more hours.

"Does it feel like something special is happening here?" Jeff asked, his eyes locked on mine.

Four days later, I approached the hostess stand at Greens Restaurant in the Marina district. "Reservation for Larsen?" I said, tugging at the hem of my clingy black minidress and hoping my wardrobe choice wasn't too bold.

"You're the first to arrive," said the hostess. "Would you like to be seated or wait here?"

"I'll wait here," I said, wanting to make sure Jeff got the full impact of my slim thirty-seven-inch-inseam legs when he arrived. "And if it's not too much trouble," I added, "I'd love to have a special table. This is our second date." I tried to appear cool and collected, but I'm sure the hostess saw right through my façade.

"I have just the table," she said. She made a notation on her seating chart and turned to greet the next customer.

I stood in the corner of the reception area and thought about the absurdity of this whirlwind courtship, of how right everything felt despite that small nagging fear within me that cautioned against expecting too much, moving too quickly. What if Jeff is just another womanizer? *He's not,* said a calm inner voice. But if he is, I silently retorted, I won't have the luxury of licking my wounds in private. Word of our personal relationship would spread throughout the workplace and my heartbreak would be public, more fodder for office gossip. So far, we'd managed to keep our personal relationship under wraps. But so far had been only four days.

Jeff entered the restaurant, automatically ducking his head a bit as though his height might be too much for the doorway. He gave me a quick kiss and we followed the hostess as she wove us through a vast open dining room with floor-to-ceiling windows looking out on the bay, the Golden Gate Bridge in the distance. The tables were rectangular and covered in white linen, but among them all was one unique table, a finely glazed cross-section of a giant redwood tree, its beauty requiring no tablecloth. It sat in the center of the restaurant as if on display.

We took our seats at that table and now we were both on display as well.

The sommelier arrived. "A bottle of Veuve Clicquot, please," Jeff said.

I'd last had this champagne a year earlier, when my girlfriend Dana and I ordered it at dinner while I was in Boston on business. After listening to my complaints about my loveless love life, Dana, for whom I'd been a bridesmaid the year before, made me write down all the attributes I was looking for in a partner. "We'll create him," she said, assuring me that I could manifest my dream man with the help of a cocktail napkin and a ballpoint pen. After dinner, she took my list home and tucked it away in a book of love poems that her husband had given her.

Moments later the sommelier returned, bottle in hand. "Is there a special occasion tonight?" he asked. Jeff pulled his gaze from my eyes and looked up at the older gentleman.

"Yes, there is," he said. Then his eyes returned to mine. "I think we may be getting engaged."

We hadn't discussed this possibility, hadn't planned on this dinner date being a time to hash out the pros and cons of spending the rest of our lives together. Yet I felt surprisingly calm as I took in Jeff's words, as if getting engaged was the most logical and natural next step for a couple who'd spent less than fourteen hours together. Any trepidation I'd had earlier was replaced by an inexplicable sense of peace, of knowing beyond doubt that this was the person I was meant to be with.

"Yes," I added, "I think we may be."

And four hours later—still seated at the table, our food virtually untouched—we were.

8

A RESPIRATION THERAPIST COMES to my room and, mercifully, removes my breathing tube. The results of the postseizure CT scan were all negative: no hemorrhaging in the brain, no fluid buildup, no apparent cause. A magnesium sulfate drip is begun to prevent further seizures.

03/11/00—Jeff talked with Dr. Osorio (whom he and everyone else are now calling Bob) and he said this seizure is simply one of the "speed bumps" in Lauren's recovery. The next speed bump is working through the pneumonia. Lauren's white count and temperature continue to be elevated.

A neurologist pays a visit to assess possible damage from my seizure last night. She shines a light in each of my eyes, her face inches from mine. I like her red hair and lilting Irish accent, though I have trouble focusing on her questions. But I like her.

She addresses Karen. "There's no pressure on her optic nerves, and no fluid there either." This is a good thing, she explains to us. She flips through my medical chart, familiarizing herself with my case. "Given all your sister has been through, a seizure is not unexpected," she says.

Soon after the neurologist leaves, a new kidney doctor appears in my room. He is tall, with thinning hair, and he wears a white lab coat like the rest of them. He has my chart in his hands and is scanning the most recent entries. I've already decided I don't like him.

"Hello, Lauren," he says, leaning over my bed.

"Listen!" I bark. "You cooperate with me and I'll cooperate with you. And if you don't, I'll kick your ass!"

I close my eyes.

"Well," he says to my sister, "that's the first time I've ever been issued an ultimatum by a patient." He addresses me again.

"Can you tell me where you are, Lauren?" he asks.

Apparently he's still here. And I'm tired of people talking to me like I'm a four-year-old. Even in my current mental state, I can recognize a patronizing tone.

"At a spa in Boulder, Colorado," I say. "Where it's *quiet*. They let us sleep here." With eyes still closed, I begin singing the words to "Rocky Mountain High." Before leaving, the kidney doctor adds his own comments to my medical chart: *Patient's lucidity weak. Keeps singing John Denver songs.*

03/11/00—Karen said she wished she had a tape recorder because Lauren is really on a wacky roll. Les, the Aussie nurse who moved to the States "in a fit of temporary insanity," whispered to Karen, "As much as she jabbers on and on, I suspect that underneath it all she's highly intelligent."

Les, the cute guy with the accent, is whispering with my sister on the other side of the room. I'm convinced that he and Karen are having an affair, and I'm concerned about what this will do to Karen's husband. It will crush him. Why is she doing this to him?

"Les!" I say, breaking up their little tryst. "It's time for me to have a shower. I *need* a shower."

Les comes to my bedside and explains that I can't have a shower because of the staples in my abdomen. I have no idea what he's talking about, no idea that even without this alleged staple issue, I'm incapable of standing, let alone showering.

"Staples in my gut, Les?" I roll my eyes and give my sister a knowing smirk.

Liz's husband stops by my room to bring her something she forgot at home. Taking his first glance at me since Clare's birth, Rick's expression is a mix of shock and forced nonchalance. He regains his composure and approaches my bed.

"I heard the doctors in the hallway saying good things about you, Lauren," he says.

"That's because I put out!" I bark. Even as the words leave my mouth I sense that I'm being inappropriate, yet I can't seem to edit my words before I speak—a side effect of encephalopathy known as disinhibition. Frustrated, I pretend not to care, and soon enough my mind moves on to a different focus.

My father-in-law and sister Steph return from their errand. Karen sent them out to find pizza for my lunch, macaroni and cheese for my dinner. She has taken on the role of my personal meal planner and she knows well my lifelong love affair with cheese. With Karen's help getting the food to my mouth, I consume one slice of vegetarian pizza and two glasses of warm orange juice.

After lunch I'm moved to a quieter room at the request of the neurologist, who wants me to get more sleep. Room 318 is at the end of the hall, six rooms away from the busy atmosphere of the nurses' station. Karen urges me to nap, but I continue to prattle on and on about things that exist in a reality to which I alone am privy.

"I want to give back to the hospital somehow," I say. "Perhaps I'll redecorate the floor above the ICU to show my gratitude." For what, I'm not sure, but before I can figure it out, my thoughts are interrupted by the steady sound of a monitor in the adjoining patient room: *Bing, bing, bing!*

"Tell the Avon lady to go away," I say. "We don't need any makeup."

"Shhhh," Karen scolds. "Try to get some rest."

I ignore her and continue talking. Using a purple marker, she writes something on a yellow notepad, then holds it up for me to read: *Shhhhhh. Wa needs to sleep. Signed, The Management.* I smile. She's funny, my sister. And I like having her here to care for me.

Karen moves to a chair in the corner of the room that she believes is beyond my line of vision. She is quiet, hopeful that I will fall asleep soon.

"I can *seeeeeeeeee* you," I say. She doesn't respond.

"I need you to call the lactation center," I say. "I want to learn how to reactivate my boobs."

Karen ignores me. I talk about my desire to breastfeed, the need for Pam's hand-me-down breast pump to be brought from home. I can't remember where I put it, but it's there somewhere. I have no concept that even if I could get milk from my now shrunken breasts, it would be contaminated. Or that Clare is living four hundred miles away. My badgering continues until Karen finally responds to one of my comments.

"I knew it!" I say. "You're there!" I am vindicated.

Karen gives up hope of getting me to sleep and pulls her chair closer so we can talk. I ask if she likes the hospital, if she likes the work she does. Yes, she tells me.

"You know," I say, fancying myself a wise career counselor, "you're very good at what you're doing. You ought to consider going into this line of work." I've forgotten that Karen has worked with patients in hospitals, nursing homes, and other institutional settings for most of her professional life. But to me, right now, all I know is that I like having her here, that it feels good to be with her. Yes, this line of work suits her well.

The following morning, I hear that Irish accent I like out in the hallway. My neurologist has returned.

"Lauren," she says kindly, "I'm going to tell you three words and I'd like you to remember them for me, okay?" She speaks quite slowly, her voice enunciating every word. I nod to show that I understand.

"Ball. Cat. House," she says. We sit in silence for ten seconds. "Can you repeat the three words to me, Lauren?"

"Ball-cat-house," I say.

"Great!" says my Irish doc.

This is stupid, I think. She jots something on her clipboard, turns to Jeff, and speaks with him for several minutes. I pay them no attention. I'm still sleepy and am having a tough time staying awake for her.

"All right, Lauren," she says, "can you still remember those three words?"

"Ball-cat-house," I say.

Again she is enthusiastic about my ability to remember them, but I'm getting bored with this game. She and Jeff continue their conversation. A few minutes pass and she asks me once more if I can remember the three words.

"Forget. Me. Not," I say.

The neurologist looks puzzled, but Jeff is reassured—a glimmer of my old self fighting back, sarcasm my weapon.

Mom and Jeff sit on opposite sides of my bed during Mom's first visit since she broke down and left the hospital five days ago. After a long stretch of silence, I turn my head toward Jeff.

"When can we fuck, hon?" I ask, having never before propositioned my husband with such profanity. My mother and husband exchange a glance.

"Did she say what I think she said?" Mom asks. Jeff nods, then turns toward me.

"Not until I know who I'm sleeping with," he says. Satisfied with his answer, I nod off again.

3/12/00 – The doctors told us to expect metabolic encephalopathy because of the giant blood clot, which creates nitrates that the liver usually takes care of. But right now, the liver is going full bore to deal with the clot and it's overwhelmed. As Lauren's ammonia level rises, so does her wackiness and the yellowness of her skin.

"Get them out!" I yell. "Use a knife and cut the bags open! They're going to kill them!"

What's wrong with these people? Can't they see all these babies? They're everywhere, trapped in plastic bags all over the floor! No one seems to care, let alone see them! I'm desperate, yet no one is helping. Jeff looks at me as if I've lost my mind. He tells me they don't exist, which only enrages me.

"Don't you see the babies?" I ask him, incredulous. I'm overwhelmed with sadness and frustration, and my face melts into tears of anguish.

"No, honey. I'm sorry, but I don't see them," he says. His voice is sad, his expression apologetic. Someone in a white lab coat enters the room.

"You!" I shout through my tears. "You're a registered certified trainer! Get the babies out and revive them!"

The white coat ignores my command, the extent of my encephalopathy well understood among the ICU staff. He huddles with my husband and mother on the other side of the room, speaking in hushed tones. When they are through, Mom returns to my bedside. Holding an imaginary pair of scissors, she tells me she sees a couple of the bags and will help free the babies inside. I turn toward Jeff with a look of smug superiority.

"See?" I say, my tone full of arrogance. "Women see things that men don't!"

Bending forward, Mom pretends to lift a bag, cut off its top. "They're not there!" I yell, my frustration now aimed at her. "They're over here!"

Again, I dissolve in tears. No one understands. Surrounded by madness, I am all alone.

The doctor in charge of the ICU decides I need to sit up in a chair. Movement will help prevent additional blood clots from forming. Offering no help, I allow Jeff and a nurse to maneuver the 250 pounds of dead weight posing as my body to a large padded chair. Others hover around, ready to help. Someone snaps a photograph of me propped up, my head leaning back and resting awkwardly against the uppermost edge of the chair, my mouth flopping open, my eyes closed.

I begin to slide down in the chair, unaware as my knees give way, collapsing me toward the floor. People grab at me, hold me in place while Jeff positions himself on a stool directly in front of me and puts his knees against mine as a barrier to prevent any further slippage. I open my eyes and survey the scene before me. There are more people than usual moving in and out of my room, more activity than I'm used to.

"This is like being in a bad B movie," I say, closing my eyes again to shut out those around me.

My "ability" to sit in the chair is rewarded with a move to the TICU, the Transitional Intensive Care Unit. It's a sign that I am improving. Compared to the stark environment of the ICU, my new room resembles a hotel. There's a television, a private bath, and a cot for overnight visitors.

I nap for two hours, but even with the extra sleep my mental acuity doesn't improve. There is more babbling, more hallucinating. Communists—anyone in a white lab coat—are trying to steal my sperm and eggs for evil purposes. They keep coming at me and it's terrifying. And now the mob is after Karen, who's been remodeling my rental home without my permission, tearing the entire roof off to add another floor but leaving the house open and unfinished. I'm petrified of how the landlords will react when they find out, and I'm so pissed at my sister for ripping my home apart that I regret cutting a deal with the mob to save her life. Confusion and sadness and anger swirl together in a hodgepodge of mixed emotions, and I'm no longer sure where one visual image stops and the next one starts. As each phantasm flies at me, I scramble to make sense of it, but some—like the brains marching up my bed—defy my interpretive abilities. In response to these images I simply scream.

At dinnertime Karen tries to feed me, placing a small bite of food on my tongue. I don't chew, so she uses her index finger to remove it. Then she pours an ounce or two of water into my mouth and all of it dribbles down my chin. One of the residents inserts a feeding tube into my left nostril, threads the tubing down into my stomach, and secures it to my face with white first-aid tape.

Hours pass, and I'm more restless than ever. I move my head rhythmically from left to right on my pillow: back and forth, back and forth, for hours, back and forth. Having been in the Transitional ICU less than eleven hours, I am evicted from my luxury room and wheeled back to the ICU.

9

A TEENAGER THUMPS HIS FOREFINGER on my belly, which looks as if I'm about to give birth to quintuplets. It makes an odd, almost hollow sound, like a bongo drum. He—this young man I don't know—has a round face, full lips, and wavy black hair. Why the hell is he thumping *my* belly? Why can't he go bug someone else? There are others surrounding my bed as well. Doctors perhaps?

Now he wants me to tell him who the president of the United States is. What a stupid question. How odd, though. I can't seem to remember who it is, so I pretend I don't hear him. The annoying teenager is actually Dr. Osorio—Bob to my family—the head of the liver transplant department, who has been closely managing my care. He doesn't push the issue of the president's identity. Instead, he asks about me.

"How does this feel?" he says, tapping his forefinger on my belly once more.

"It hurts," I say. He stops tapping.

"Does your abdomen feel tight?"

"Very," I say. "And it still hurts."

"Gas," he says.

Looking more closely at his face, I realize he's not a teenager at all. He's a grown man, even has a few gray hairs. He has a gentle way about him and he looks kind, so I decide I like him, especially now that he has stopped drumming his fingers on my stomach.

"Lauren, do you know what happened to you?"

I'm embarrassed because it feels as if I ought to know the answer to this one. But I don't. Again I pretend not to hear the question. Interpreting my silence as a no, he tells me about the baby, the liver failure, the seizure, and the blood transfusions. *Blood transfusions! I'll bet I have AIDS now!* I immediately think of that article I read years ago about a boy—was his name Ryan?—who contracted AIDS from a blood transfusion and was then banned from school, his family taunted. I remember another article about him years later, his face gracing the cover of *People* magazine. He had died. *I'm screwed.*

"We can relieve some of that pressure in your abdomen," Bob says. "It's called paracentesis, or a belly tap. We'll remove some of the fluid that's built up in there and that'll take the pressure off everything else. It'll make you much more comfortable." He mentions that my sonogram results from this morning showed large pockets of fluid—mostly dead hemorrhaged blood—in my abdomen, confirmation that I need paracentesis. He does not mention that a six-inch needle the width of an ice pick is the primary tool used to perform the procedure.

"Michael will do the belly tap," he continues, looking toward a twenty-something man on the other side of my bed. It's the Middle Eastern guy, the one I remember not liking for some reason. Only now, I realize he's not my roommate as I thought before. I'm still not sure I like him.

The group of lab coats surrounding me disperses, leaving only Jeff and Peter, one of my regular nurses. A half hour passes and Michael returns. The young doctor speaks to me as if we've had many conversations before, so I pretend to re-member him. His manner reminds me of my early professional days at PepsiCo, its marketing cubicles overflowing with cocky young MBAs. Like me when I was in my twenties, Michael is quick-witted and self-assured, but seems devoid of the com-passion and empathy that comes from personal experience with suffering.

"First, we're going to numb the area with lidocaine," he says, brushing a cold liquid on my belly. "It's a topical anesthetic."

"What about additional pain medication?" Jeff asks.

"She won't need it," says Michael. "She won't feel much once this settles in." The shift in Peter's expression tells me he disagrees with the young doctor's assessment.

Michael turns toward the tray of sterile implements he set down by my bed when he entered. I try not to notice the huge needle he picks up. I also try not to notice that as he begins the procedure, Jeff purposely turns away.

"Okay, Lauren, this is going to feel like a bee sting," Michael says. He plunges the thick needle into the right side of my belly.

"Ow!" I snap. I've been stung by a bee before and this feels nothing like that. Jeff turns toward me and winces. Always my protector, I know he would take all of these medical assaults for me if he could. At this point in my illness, I would gladly let him. As the needle goes deeper into my belly, I groan, squeeze my eyes shut tight. Perhaps if I can't see it, I won't feel it.

"You shouldn't be feeling this," says Michael.

"But I do!" I say, opening my eyes and glaring at him. I'm hell-bent on hiding my vulnerability from this young doctor, ten years my junior, but the tears are already welling up, so I mask my pain with confrontation.

"I'll bet you've never had a belly tap," I say. Michael smirks. He thinks I'm joking. If I could, I would punch him right now.

Peter stands at Michael's side holding a clear plastic bag that's connected to plastic tubing on the end of the needle, which remains—painfully—lodged in my abdomen. The bag is filling up with a murky fluid, like curdled milk mixed with brownish-red blood. I hear them conferring with one another, tossing little phrases about my progress back and forth: *Okay, we're good; almost full. Okay, switch.* Another one-liter bag is attached and filling steadily. Peter caps off the first bag and places it on the countertop by the sink. Jeff steps toward the bag and examines it.

"Gross," he says.

Again there is conferring between doctor and nurse, and another bag is filled and swapped out. Then another. And another. Four liters of gunk—roughly nine pounds' worth—have been extracted from my belly. Michael removes the needle and shoots me a know-it-all smile. "That wasn't so bad, was it?" he says. He peels off his thin sterile gloves and drops them in the medical waste bin by the sink.

"Piece of cake," I say. *Asshole.*

03/15/00—The Rational Period begins. Jeff spent the night with Lauren. At 1 a.m. an IV line had been threaded in through the tube in Lauren's jugular vein. Lauren joked the entire time. Her kidneys aren't doing well, but this is expected when there's been liver failure. The liver can shut down the kidneys, but the kidneys can't shut down the liver. This is known as hepatorenal syndrome.

One of the renal specialists tells Jeff—and me, though I'm not paying much attention—that my kidneys present the biggest challenge right now. Lab work indicates an abnormality, but the reason is unclear. It could be from the dopamine they gave me early on to "open up" my kidneys, he explains. Or it could be from all the Lasix I was given to curb the fluid retention. Could be that there's not enough fluid in the blood vessels. Or that there's too much bilirubin, which acts as a toxin to the kidneys. Or that the antibiotic I'm on for the pneumonia I developed has caused a reaction.

In other words, nobody knows why.

My nurses watch for signs of urine moving through the Foley catheter that runs from my urinary tract to a bag hanging off the bed. Any urine is good urine. It means my kidneys are still working, albeit poorly.

"There's a bit!" says a nurse. I look at the catheter line. There is nothing resembling pee moving through it. Instead, a thick brown mud—more like coffee grounds, really—inches its way through the clear tube. I should be shocked, but at this point the whole experience is so bizarre that I find myself taking on the perspective of a curious outsider, detached from this science experiment that my body has become.

There's a knock at the door and a medical technician wheels in a large cart holding a portable dialysis machine. She hooks me up to it, using the port that was implanted in my chest sometime while I was either well sedated or unconscious, probably both. I don't remember the acquisition of this odd little medical device, but now that it's being put to use I take a closer look. Two inches by two inches in size, it resembles a computer plug, the kind that connects the CPU to the printer. But unlike a computer system, this plug connects directly to flesh. *My* flesh.

A nurse brings a stack of warm blankets into the room and explains that dialysis often makes patients cold. She pulls back my covers and puts two warm blankets directly on my body, then pulls the other covers up again, gently tucking me in as if I'm a child and it's bedtime. These small acts of nurturing performed regularly by my nurses provide the emotional sustenance I need to keep from completely falling apart over what has become my life, the vast schism between my carefully devised plans and my current reality.

The dialysis machine is turned on and I'm surprised by how noisy it is. I close my eyes and pretend that the thumping and whirring of the machine is actually something soothing, perhaps waves crashing on the ocean's shoreline. A portion of my blood is sucked out of my body and into the machine, where it is stripped of toxins. Then the clean blood is pumped back into my body. This happens over and over again, and the entire process takes about three hours. I feel a deep internal chill the entire time despite the heaping on of more warm blankets every fifteen minutes. But I don't mind because dialysis doesn't hurt, and I'm grateful for this stretch of time without pain.

Within hours my kidneys are producing an abundance of dark yellow urine. My doctors and nurses are pleased because this means the dialysis was effective. By clearing the blood of excessive toxins, my kidneys are better able to do their job. But by the next morning my urinary output is still not exceeding, or even matching, my fluid input, so the dialysis machine is wheeled back into my room. The doctors seem to view dialysis as a serious procedure, not without risks and not to be taken lightly. Too much dialysis can prevent the kidneys from working on their own again, necessitating a kidney transplant. I, however, love dialysis. During the lengthy treatments nothing else can be done to me, except for the occasional temperature-taking. The average ICU patient requires 178 individual actions per day, but dialysis offers a reprieve from this onslaught. No poking, no prodding, no rolling.

As my blood is cleared of impurities so too is my brain. My mental capacity is best immediately following dialysis. Pam sits with me after my second three-hour procedure and we talk like the old days in graduate school when we hung around the third-floor student lounge between classes. With a clear mind, I no longer wonder if I've had two babies or three. It's one. And her name is Clare. And she's fifteen days old. And she's living four hundred miles away.

"I feel like I've deserted her," I say.

Pam doesn't shush me or disagree or try to change the subject. As the mother of two-year-old twins born of a difficult pregnancy, she can empathize. Like me, career came first for her after we graduated together from UCLA's MBA program twelve years ago. But eventually her eighty-hour workweeks at the Walt Disney Company were replaced with decorating a nursery in Disney characters and stockpiling CDs of Disney sing-along songs. All the passion Pam had put into being a corporate executive was shifted into being a mom.

"I get that Clare's better off with Tim and De right now," I say. "But that doesn't make me feel any better about it." Pam's silence tells me she understands, and I pass another sleepless night with my friend.

03/17/00—Lauren is uncomfortable. She doesn't have much of an appetite and it's so noisy in the ICU she hasn't been able to sleep well. Tim made tollhouse cookies for her to try and pique her appetite. Jeff is near the breaking point.

My belly, though softer after the paracentesis procedure two days ago, is once again tight. The pain is immense, any shift of my body causing an electric current to run through my abdomen. It began as I ate a small breakfast after Pam left this morning. The head of the ICU explains that I'm suffering from gas pains, which can be quite debilitating given my other medical circumstances.

Someone gives me a pill to swallow and within minutes I feel woozy. I'm told to tilt my head back and open my mouth as wide as possible. I'm not told to close my eyes, but I do this anyway, not wanting to see what comes next, my gag reflex on alert despite the medication. A tube is put in my mouth and slowly pushed down my throat. I struggle against the desire to vomit, willing myself to relax, my breathing labored by the partial blockage. The tube reaches my stomach and the sensation of it creeping down my throat stops. The other end of the tube is attached to a machine on a cart by my bed, and with the flip of a switch the sound of the machine drowns out the sound of my gagging. Gas is sucked out of my stomach and bowels, and minutes later the machine is turned off, the tube pulled quickly from my throat. I take a deep breath and think it's over.

But it's not.

Michael enters my room, a tray of paracentesis tools in his hands. *Not again,* I think, willing myself not to cry. Another belly tap, another huge needle, and four more liters of dead blood—nine more pounds of poison—are removed. My abdomen is once again softer and the gas pains are gone, but I'm physically and emotionally drained. Without the benefit of encephalopathy, I'm now acutely aware of every invasive medical procedure in this odyssey called survival.

Unable to sleep, I decide to try reading. The last time I read a book I was pregnant and sure about the future. Now I only look pregnant and am sure of nothing.

Given the day's activities thus far, along with the feeling of *Why me?* that has crept into my psyche, I'm in need of some inspiration. As I've done for years, I close my eyes and lift the cover of *Simple Abundance*, the book I'd asked Jeff to retrieve from home earlier today. Allowing the pages to fall open to whatever I'm "meant" to read, I let my finger drift across both open pages until it comes to rest where it wants, my assumption being that these are the words most pertinent to my current situation. I open my eyes, look at the sentence my finger is pointing to, and laugh. It reads: *Whatever situation exists in your life right now, accept it.*

If there is a god, he, she, or it has one hell of a sense of humor. I continue reading. *Cast a glance around and acknowledge what's going on. This is what is really happening in my life at the present moment. This is okay. This is real life.*

I skip to another paragraph. *Before we can change anything in our life we have to recognize that this is the way it's meant to be right now.* The relevance of these words stuns me, and a sense of fate creeps into my psyche. Is this all part of some cosmic plan, a plan far grander and more significant than any of the myriad one-year, five-year, and ten-year plans I've crafted over the years? Could my more religious friends be right, that there is a predetermined purpose to my life?

Before I can delve too deeply into the philosophical undercurrents of my illness, the physical realities of my circumstances pull me back. My arms begin to weaken from holding the book upright. Resting it on top of my belly is out of the question, as is turning on my side, so I skip to the last paragraph.

Today, let go of the struggle. Allow the healing process of change to begin. You're ready to move on.

You're goddamned right I am! I set the book on my bedside table and close my eyes. With a level of optimism reminiscent of the old Lauren, I know with certainty that I can do this for another day.

10

AMY IS YOUNG, MID-TWENTIES PERHAPS, and has a fresh face and petite frame. Cradling her clipboard, she looks like she's playing dress-up in her green scrubs and white lab coat. I have always imagined physical therapists to be massive muscular men, tough yet affable. I can't imagine tiny sweet Amy maneuvering my six-one, two-hundred-plus-pound body through various physical therapy exercises.

"Okay, Lauren," she says, her expression one of complete optimism, "we're going to get you out of bed today." I stifle a chuckle. I know beyond a doubt that this body is not going to stand, not today.

I first met Amy a few days ago. After brief introductions, she pulled back my covers and asked me to lift my right leg about six inches in the air. I looked at my right leg and willed it to rise, but it didn't move.

"How about the left one?" she asked. I couldn't move that one either.

"Well, let's just try rolling them side to side. Can you do that?" she asked. I was impressed with her unflappable belief in me. I looked at my legs again, willed them to roll side to side. They did and I was pleased, even proud.

But getting out of bed? Today? No way.

"I can't," I tell her. I don't even pretend to try. I hold her gaze and she knows I'm not joking. I will not walk today. She's wiser than I've given her credit for because she doesn't fight me on this point.

"Okay, then. How about we just sit up?"

With more trepidation than I'm willing to admit, I agree to give it a try. Amy summons one of the nurses to help as she pulls back the blankets covering my legs. Jeff gets up from his chair on the other side of the room, sets his book down, and moves in to watch, ready to help—or intervene on my behalf— if need be. Using the controls on the arm railing, Amy raises the back of my bed to its uppermost position. Though still reclined, I'm more upright than I've been in weeks. So far so good. She takes hold of my hands while a nurse positions herself to prop me up from behind.

"On three," Amy says, and begins to count. At three, I am slowly hoisted into a full sitting-up position, and my equilibrium wanes the more vertical I become.

"Deep breaths, Lauren," says the nurse, her strong arms supporting my back. "Just keep breathing and the nausea will pass."

How did she know I feel like I'm about to hurl? She rubs my back while holding me in place. Again, I experience that feeling I've had on numerous occasions since regaining mental clarity—nurses get it. There is something about their demeanor that makes me feel both nurtured and understood. Sure, there are one or two nurses with whom I don't feel a connection, like Bella, whom I've privately nicknamed Bella Lugosi. But mostly they are like Peter, whose dead-on impersonation of a Russian spy kept my family both amused and sane during my Communist-plot hallucinations. Or Carol, whom I don't remember from the first hospital, but who shows up every couple of days to sit with me. Or this one, who seems to instinctively understand how comforting the simple gesture of rubbing my back is right now.

"Don't look down, Lauren. Just keep looking into my eyes," Amy says. I do as she tells me and begin to feel more stable, as she and the nurse continue holding me in place. A few minutes pass this way and Amy asks Jeff to take her place holding my hands. She carefully scoops my thick edematous legs into her arms and guides them to the side of the bed. Jeff and the nurse rotate my body as Amy hangs my legs off the mattress. She gives me a thumbs-up, as if I've just crossed the finish line of a marathon. Through labored breathing, I smile. So does Jeff. All of us are fully aware of what a huge accomplishment this is. We remain like this for five minutes, Jeff and the nurse holding me up, and me, just proud to be held in place.

"Want to try a chair?" Amy asks.

"Sure," I say, my confidence running strong.

Amy drags the large padded chair in the corner next to the bed. She puts a large disposable pad, akin to a diaper, on the seat. With my rectal catheter removed and little control over my bowels, there's no telling when something will slip out. Better safe than soiled.

"Okay, let's give it a try," Amy says, trading places with the nurse. "Jeff, you take that side, I'll take this side, and on three we'll lift her to standing." Jeff nods his agreement, and they each move into position, tightening their grip on my upper arms, which are full of marble-sized knots from a profusion of injections over the past weeks. On three, I feel myself rising to standing position, albeit stooped, for the first time in eighteen days. Jeff and Amy strain to hold me up. The nurse quickly maneuvers the chair closer to my backside as Jeff and Amy rotate my body, my feet still firmly planted on the floor. In this hunched position, my flimsy hospital gown falls forward, revealing two enormous dark bruises that run from my armpits to my thighs and partway around my back, another side effect of the massive hemorrhage.

"Hold on," says the nurse, and she lifts the disposable pad, stacks two thick pillows on the chair and places the pad on top of them. "This should help soften things for those bruises."

On three, they lower me onto the pillows, and the nurse stuffs an additional pillow behind my back to support what remains of my posture. I sit here, uncomfortable but still proud, for an hour and fifteen minutes.

By midday, I'm back in my hospital bed. A lunch tray is set on my over-table, but I'm afraid to eat, afraid that the severe gas pains I experienced yesterday will return, that I'll need another belly tap, another tube shoved down my throat. Jeff knows better than to push the issue. Instead, he reads to me from Rachel Remen's new book, a collection of stories from her medical practice. Jeff is a fabulous reader, his voice as smooth and rich as the day I first heard it four years ago, his ability to pace a story well-honed from his early career as a public radio news anchor. I am comforted to hear about the hardships of others, especially knowing that many of them survived. The theme running through the book is not one of unbridled optimism and forced positive thinking, but grace in the face of life's unexpected challenges. Seldom have I so connected with a book's message. I close my eyes and allow Jeff's narration to cocoon me with empathy.

Later that afternoon, the dialysis cart is wheeled into my room for another round of blood cleansing. Afterward a blood sample is taken for my twice-daily lab tests. The results are disheartening. My clotting factors are too low, my bilirubin too high. My liver is still only partially working and my incision from the two surgeries seems to be leaking blood into my abdomen. Again, the experts are stumped as to why. Mom, who flew home several days ago for a break, boards another plane back to San Francisco.

03/21/00—Karen had a dream last night. In it, we family members were at the shore. We went into the ocean and ended up treading water to stay afloat. Not Lauren. She was riding on the crest of the waves, reciting lines. Karen's interpretation is that Lauren knows what she has to do; we're just there to support her.

The Ativan I was given to help me sleep doesn't work, so I pass the night talking with John, the Hispanic nurse who left the fur coat business, he tells me, to find work that fed his soul. Nursing suits him, and he's fast becoming one of my favorites. When he ducks out of my room to tend to his other patient, I stare at the clock on the wall, hoping the slight ticking sound of the second hand will steer my thoughts away from the questions that have begun to haunt me on nights like this. Did complacency cause me to miss the warning signs? Worse yet, did I do something to cause this? Memories of earlier excesses in my life bombard my senses, such as the frequency with which I drank alcohol in high school and college, assuming that everyone was doing it. And when I worked long hours in the soft-drink industry, I drank four to six Diet Pepsis each day. That couldn't have helped my liver either. And what of all those Taco Bell meals I ate, almost daily, throughout my pregnancy? Didn't I know that a thirty-two-ounce soda and all that fast food would surely take its toll? *What the hell was I thinking?*

I wasn't thinking. That's the problem. I was cruising through life on optimism at its extreme: denial. It couldn't happen to me, wouldn't happen to me. But it did. And now there's a baby out there who doesn't know her parents, a baby who would be better off with a different mother, one with less guilt gnawing at her conscience.

Noticing that I'm still awake at four, John asks me if I'd like to try sitting up again, this time on a commode, which looks like a combination high chair and toilet. This will allow him to clean both me and my bed sheets, he explains, which surely will make me feel better. Reluctantly, I agree.

Although considerably shorter than me, John is strong and needs no additional help to pivot me from bed to commode. His face is inches from mine as he hoists me from under my arms. His breath is stale and I try hard not to let it show in my facial expression. I have no idea that my own breath is exponentially worse, my throat still coated with an infection called thrush, my teeth unbrushed since Clare's birth. I sit on the commode as John changes my sheets, regaling me with stories of his life. Then he hoists me back into the bed, where I drift off from the exhaustion of simply having been moved.

When I awaken, Mom is sitting across the room, reading glasses on, book in hand, head tilted forward. It's a familiar pose I've seen in numerous settings throughout my life: at nighttime in her bed when I was a kid growing up in New Jersey; over the holidays by the fireplace in Houston after she met and married my stepdad; during happy hour in her Boulder living room after she and John retired there. Seldom in life had I seen my mother without a book within arm's reach, and as long as I can remember she's been a voracious reader. I let a minute pass before interrupting her and when I do, I break completely from our family's norms of communication.

"I really love you, Mom," I say. "I'm sorry I'm taking you away from John, but I really appreciate everything you're doing. Thanks for being here for me."

For only the second time in my life, I see my mother cry.

Lunch arrives and today I'm willing to eat. The doctors believe my previous gas pains were caused by one of the many medications, which they've discontinued. I'm helped onto the commode and it is here where I consume a purposely bland meal: half a peanut butter sandwich, a few apple slices, a small bowl of Jell-O cubes, and an eight-ounce carton of Resource. Mom sits with me while I feed myself. When my bowels suddenly get noisy and evacuate their contents into the portable toilet bowl beneath me, she doesn't miss a beat.

"Garbage in, garbage out," she deadpans, and we both laugh.

A nurse removes the soiled toilet bowl and replaces it with a clean one. I push my lunch tray aside, no longer hungry. Mom begins to brush my greasy hair, pulling it off my face and into a loose ponytail. It's been decades since she styled my hair for me, and style was never a guarantee.

"I don't want to look like the kids in *The Brady Bunch*," I say, thinking back on her infamous "water spout" hairdos of the late sixties. She laughs and sets the brush down. She begins gently massaging my shoulders and upper back. We are both quiet as she does this, but after a few minutes I break the silence. Still half-naked and seated on the commode, I ask, "Are we having quality time, Mom?"

Later that afternoon, Amy stops by and once more I'm roused from my bed. "This time," my physical therapist says, "we're going to walk."

I know I can't put her off forever, so I acquiesce without an argument. Someone slides slippers onto my feet. Once I'm in standing position, a walker is put in front of me. Amy firmly holds my right upper arm, a nurse the left one. Another nurse pushes my IV pole and Mom holds my urine bag. With my entourage of four, I slowly shuffle toward the hallway, each leg feeling like it has a concrete block tied to it, each forward movement painstakingly slow.

"Look straight ahead, not down," counsels Amy.

"Lauren, are you okay?" asks Mom. "You look like you might pass out."

"I'm okay," I say. My voice is strained, as if I'm a weight lifter struggling to hold an inordinately heavy dumbbell over my head. "Just a little dizzy."

When I make it to the doorway, a full twelve feet from where I began, Amy tells me I can turn around, that this is enough for my first time. If I could, I would hug her right now. Instead, I pause to catch my breath and take in all the activity outside my room.

One of my regular nurses walks down the hallway toward me and stops dead in her tracks when she sees me, her hands flying reflexively to her mouth as her eyes widen in surprise.

"Look at you go!" she says. She is beaming. So am I. Bravado consumes me.

"You watch me walk tomorrow," I say, still winded. "I've got a child to raise."

As I pivot back toward my bed, I see that she's crying. Retracing my steps, I keep my gaze focused on the goal: my bed. I'm nauseous and exhausted and need to lie down again.

But inside I'm looking to the heavens, pumping my fist skyward in victory.

II

MY TWENTY-FOUR-FOOT WALK yesterday earned me a transfer back to the Transitional ICU, Room 335. It's nice—still a hospital room, but much larger and better furnished than the rooms of the surgical ICU. With my newfound sense of sanity I now care about my surroundings, wanting them to be as pleasant and healing as possible. Sabra made several affirmation signs that now hang on the walls. *Everything works in harmony to heal me* reads one. *I am stronger each day!* and *I am healed!* hang closest to my bed. And to affirm my ability to get enough rest, the last sign reads *I sleep with ease.* When Mom sees this one she says, "Who's Ease? Is he cute?"

Jeff brought some things from home to decorate my new room. A framed photo of Spike sits on top of the plain lightwood armoire. A small gold sun ornament hangs overhead. Photos of Clare with my brother, his wife, and their children grace the walls. She's such a pretty little baby, I think as I survey the photos. But she looks sad, almost as if she's searching for something. Or someone. Or am I just projecting?

On another wall is a collage of twelve photos from my wedding day, all of them taken during our first dance, a professionally choreographed number Jeff and I had secretly learned to surprise and amuse our guests. As I look at those photos, I remember how nervous and giddy I was as the live orchestra moved from the calm rhythm of "You Stepped Out of a Dream" toward its crescendo, and Jeff and I broke into our one-of-a-kind dance moves—twirling, swaying, bobbing, even monkey-walking—before returning to the steady flow of a fox-trot. As the final note of the song approached, Jeff dipped me back until my shoulder-length hair grazed the ground, my left leg pointing up toward a canopy of redwood trees. It would really suck if he drops me, I remember thinking at the time. He didn't, and the crowd—more than a hundred of our closest friends—went wild, clapping and cheering.

I used to look at these photos and wish I'd had my hair professionally styled that day, or think my hips were too wide for the cut of that dress. Now I look at them and see two people whose auras are shouting with joy and silliness and possibility as they laugh their way through their first dance as husband and wife, and I think How wonderful to have a body that works!

An eight-by-ten-inch photo of me at the Los Angeles Marathon hangs on one door of the armoire, directly in my line of sight. Even after running more than twenty-six miles over four-and-a-half hours, I looked strong as I crossed the finish line. My outfit—running shorts, tank top, and visor—was neon pink so my friends on the sidelines could spot me in the field of 18,000 runners. My tank top had my name in large black iron-on lettering, so those who didn't know me could cheer for me too. I was never shy about asking for encouragement during a marathon, that particular race being my second of six. I decided to run my first marathon when my friend Carol and I were vacationing in Italy after college. Over a carafe of cheap Chianti, we each wrote out a list titled Things I Want to Do Before I Die. On mine, among other things, was: get married, learn to speak a foreign language, run a 10K. Carol scrutinized my list.

"A 10K?" she asked. "You can do better than that." She thought a moment and then said, "I know! Let's run a *marathon* together!"

So we did. New York City, November 1988. Carol almost dropped out when she hit the wall at mile twenty. I prodded her to keep going and we crossed the finish line together, her marathon career ending right then and there. I felt like hell and limped for a week, but I was hooked.

How wonderful to have a body that works.

Mom hoists me from the bed and assists me with a stand-and-pivot maneuver onto the commode, where I stay for half an hour waiting for my bowels to move. They seem to have a mind of their own, so I'm never sure when they're going to evacuate. Just as surprising is what comes out. It's nothing that resembles normal—or even abnormal—poop, a fact I find more fascinating than disturbing. This is not my body. It belongs to the sick woman who has taken my place, so how can I take any of these biological oddities personally?

When I'm ready to return to bed, Mom moves into position once more. "On three," she says, having adopted the common hospital approach. But on three, I remain where I am. I have nothing left to give, and my current weight is too much for my mother to handle alone. I force myself to laugh about it when, truly, I want to cry. Yesterday I walked. Today I can do nothing.

Mom leaves to find help, and a few minutes later two muscular twenty-something men in standard-issue blue scrubs—the Lift Team, as they're called—enter my room. Both tall and handsome, these are the kind of guys I could have, and most likely would have, seduced in my younger days. They pull me to standing and pivot my large stooped form. As before, my hospital gown falls forward, revealing most of my naked body, including the ghastly grape-sized hemorrhoids I discovered when I stood for the first time two days ago. Under normal circumstances, I'd be mortified that these young men are seeing me this way. But these aren't normal circumstances, and I don't give it a second thought.

03/22/00—Just before 5 p.m., Lauren felt a little nauseated and dizzy. Later in the evening, she vomited. They think it may have been due to an anti-nausea medication. Go figure.

Mom and Jeff return to my room together after a coffee break and find me depressed. "What's wrong, hon?" Jeff asks.

"I feel like I'm screwing up everyone's life with this stupid illness," I say, crying. They look at each other and seem to communicate telepathically. Linking arms, they begin singing "Side by Side," which our eight young nieces, nephews, and godchildren sang during our wedding ceremony.

"Through all kinds of weather, what if the sky should fall?" Mom and Jeff croon, their legs kicking in unison, first to the left, then to the right. "Just as long as we're together, it won't matter at all."

Their silliness does nothing to improve my mood, but the two of them look as happy as a couple of four-year-olds stomping through a mud puddle after a storm. I can't begrudge them this small reprieve of goofiness. Their song complete, Jeff leans over my bed, pulls off his wedding ring, and points to the inscription: *Side by Side.*

"See that?" he says. "Don't worry about what this is or isn't doing to others. Just get better."

It would not be possible for me to love my husband more than I do at this moment.

After another round of in-room dialysis, Peter stops by. I don't remember much from the many times he helped me in the ICU, but he and Mom talk like old friends. Clearly, he has won her approval and that's enough for me. Since my move two days ago, I'm no longer his patient. Yet here he is, spending his coffee break with us. Mom complains to him about the nurses' aides in the Transitional ICU waking me to check my vital signs, despite the prominent sign on my door that says I'm not to be disturbed if I'm sleeping.

"Some of them have IQs equal to the room temperature," says Peter. Mom laughs, and I suspect it is his wit that made Peter her favorite nurse. He shares stories of his other patients, many of them older and not doing well. At the request of the patients' families, everyone in the ICU is working hard to keep them alive long enough for other family members to arrive so that they can say their goodbyes.

"It's like rearranging deck chairs on the *Titanic,*" he says. Another smile from Mom. And a realization by me: Perhaps Peter is here not only to comfort my mother but also to comfort himself. Perhaps the constant threat of death that permeates the work of an intensive-care nurse must be counterbalanced with the promise offered by a patient who actually pulls through. Perhaps this is the real reason for Peter's visit.

03/23/00—The doctors said Lauren is still at a plateau in her recovery—getting neither better nor worse.

"I'm giving the doctors one more week to get me better," I tell Jeff, trying to make my withered voice sound as forceful as possible. "If they can't do it by then, I'm going home and doing it my way."

I hand him the action plan I wrote at four this morning during another mostly sleepless night. Tired and frustrated, I decided to take charge of my recovery. Jeff looks at the piece of paper, titled simply PLAN. The handwriting is light and spidery, not at all like my usual firm confident penmanship. *Wind down all drugs by end of month*, it begins. *Hospital bed at home, oxygen, no heavy physical therapy to restart bleeding.* Then the list takes a definite shift, moving into a variety of alternative approaches I want to try: *Meditation, aromatherapy, music therapy, white healing lights, acupuncture, gentle massage.*

"Okay," says Jeff. He neither encourages nor discourages me. He doesn't ask how I intend to leave the hospital when I can barely walk even with assistance. He simply acknowledges that I have made this list, and his acknowledgment is enough for me.

My next round of lab work reveals that my "numbers," as the docs like to call them, continue to be off and that my white blood cell count is elevated once more, a common indicator of infection. More antibiotics are added to my growing regimen of daily pharmaceuticals, as infections are a risk not worth taking. When my pills arrive, I question the nurse about each one, my desire for control growing by the day.

"What's this one?" I say, picking up a dark green capsule from the small white paper cup.

"It's Actigall," says the nurse.

"What's it for?"

"It prevents bile stones from forming. Pretty common for liver failure patients." There is not a trace of annoyance or impatience in her voice, even though the number of patients she is responsible for in the TICU is twice that of the ICU nurses. I take the pill.

"What about this one?" I ask, now holding up a pink-and-blue capsule.

"Zinc sulfate," she says. "Helps balance the chemicals in your body." I take the pill.

"And this?"

"Titralac. Helps prevent bone loss due to inactivity." God knows I've been inactive. I take the pill.

Our conversation continues like this for a good five minutes: me dipping an unsteady hand into the paper cup and with shaky fingers pulling out one pill at a time, turning to the nurse, and awaiting an explanation before taking each. It takes more time this way, but she seems to understand the importance of my need to control the process. Partway through, I drop a pill. My nurse searches for it in the folds of my bed linens, then takes my wobbly right hand and places the pill on my palm, gently folding my fingers around it so I can put it in my mouth myself. This small act of respect is performed with such reverence I must look away to prevent my tears from flowing.

03/24/00—Les, the Aussie RN, stopped by while Lauren was sleeping. Said it was nice to see the support of such a loving family and friends. He also said we shouldn't become fixated on Lauren's monitors, numbers, tests, etc., that they're intended for the hospital staff. He encouraged us to focus instead on the love and support of family, friends, and staff.

A nurse enters my room holding an exquisite bouquet of roses. She sets them on the bedside table and Mom picks up the card.

"It says *Our thoughts are with you.* Signed *Membership Directors Keith Moore and Betty Sayler and all of us at the San Francisco Tennis Club.*" I laugh out loud.

"What's so funny?" she asks.

"We paid a small fortune to join that club three months ago after Jeff sold his company," I explain. "Went there maybe seven times max since then." I tell Mom how much the initiation fees and monthly dues are and she furrows her brow, doing calculations in her head.

"That's about four hundred dollars a visit!" she says, "They should've sent you a whole *truckload* of roses!"

She moves the flowers to the windowsill next to the bouquet that arrived earlier from Jeff's employer. There's another knock at the door and the same nurse returns, this time a huge gift basket in her arms.

"Someone's popular," she says.

"Jesus!" says Mom, surveying the basket, which is two feet in diameter and filled with flowers, Brie, fruit, crackers, and chocolate-covered almonds. Except for the fruit, none of the gourmet treats appeal to my altered taste buds, but I'm touched nonetheless. Mom pulls the card off the outer cellophane wrapper and reads it to herself. This time, it is she who laughs.

"What?" I ask. "Who's it from?"

"There's no signature!" she says. She pulls the ribbons and cellophane off the basket, digs through its contents and finds nothing to indicate who sent it. Regardless, she pops a grape into her mouth.

"I suppose all this is *one* benefit of getting sick," I say.

"You have no idea," Mom says. "We turned away dozens of floral arrangements and balloon bouquets before this, sent them all down to the children's ward because we couldn't have them in the ICU."

"Wow," I say.

It has been, and will remain, a small and protective team of family and friends who are permitted to interact with me directly. Anyone outside this tight-knit group can only participate in peripheral ways: the meal preparation system that Sabra's sister organized to feed my family, blood donations made in my honor, gifts that began showing up at our home on the third day, when news of Clare's imminent discharge from the hospital spread and our friend Roxanna left a large basket filled with baby supplies—bottles, soy formula, diapers, wipes, diaper rash cream, and blankets—on our doorstep with a card that read *Hang in there*. I'm more touched by these kindnesses than I let on, allowing myself only the briefest pauses to reflect on all the goodness others have shown me. As if bobbing in the middle of the ocean with a life ring, I'm no longer drowning, but not yet safely to shore. I must preserve what little energy I have, keeping a laser-like focus on the destination, fearful that if I stop too long to appreciate the beauty that surrounds me I may drown in a sea of gratitude.

12

DURING MORNING ROUNDS, we learn that my liver values have been rising over the past several days. Mom hears this and is relieved until Bob tells us that higher values are bad, lower values good.

"Then why the hell do they call them *values?*" she mutters to no one in particular.

Turning his attention to me, Bob says, "I'm afraid we need to do another liver biopsy." I nod to indicate my understanding, when in fact I have no idea what I'm in for: that I'll be wide awake for the procedure; that I'm still far too bloated for the doctors to get to my liver through my abdomen; that they'll remove five tiny pieces of my liver by going in through my neck. During the first transjugular biopsy eighteen days ago, I had the benefit of being semicomatose. Today, I have no such luck.

These liver samples are needed to run additional tests to check for genetic problems, autoimmune disorders, or other clues as to why my body isn't recovering. Specialists in various fields are consulting on my case from different areas of the country: a preeclampsia expert in Mississippi; a fatty-liver expert in Missouri; and a handful of researchers from the Mayo Clinic in Minnesota. There is little agreement among those treating me, a reality that both disheartens and infuriates me.

Mom encourages Jeff to take a break, maybe go for a walk. She'll stay with me throughout the procedure, she reassures him. He looks at me as if trying to gauge my current level of need. Over the past three weeks, my reliance on—and at times, demand for—Jeff's presence has been fairly constant, save for the days my sister Karen has been in town. Only recently have I begun to grasp the toll this experience is taking on him. I see it in his furrowed brow as he flips through my medical chart, checking the latest blood test results, the empty look that's replaced his usual certitude, the way he now mechanically deals with others. An atheist, Jeff has no god from whom to consciously draw strength. Nature, fresh air, the great outdoors—these are his religion.

"Go ahead, hon," I say, "I'll be fine," though as the words leave my mouth I'm not sure I believe them. With greater awareness of those around me, I've been trying to expand my perspective to include what their needs might be. Yet most of my focus is still centered on *my* needs and *my* fears, and in a sense I can tell I'm now testing Jeff's loyalty. He kisses me goodbye, then turns to go, and a pang of disappointment grips my chest.

Three members of the Lift Team enter my room and push a gurney adjacent to my hospital bed, snapping the wheel brakes in place with their feet. One of them takes his position at my feet, one at my upper body, and the other at my abdomen. Mom hovers around to make sure they're gentle with me.

"On three," says the one in the middle, reaching across the center of the gurney and slowly sliding his arms under my backside. Any sort of movement still hurts, though no longer unbearably so. Once I'm on the gurney, Mom fusses with my hospital gown, pillows, and blankets. She understands how sensitive my body is to the smallest things: the bunching up of sheets underneath my midsection, the pillow under my head that isn't positioned just right. She pulls and tucks and smoothes until I'm content. I like this feeling—that of a small child, nurtured and safe. I'm with my mommy and she'll take care of me. I give little thought to the idea that *I* am a mommy now, that it is *I* who should be taking care of my own small child.

Mom walks alongside the gurney as I'm wheeled out of the Transitional ICU and down to the surgical wing of the hospital, where the operating rooms are linked like boxcars on a freight train. We wait alone in what appears to be a conference room across the hall from our scheduled OR. It has one whole wall of large windows looking out on a perfect San Francisco afternoon. The sun is bright and its direct angle on this side of the building has warmed the room considerably. It feels good to bask in such warmth and blinding light as I lie on my gurney, awaiting the arrival of the liver biopsy specialist.

"Would you mind doing some energy work on me?" I ask Mom. She's not a trained alternative healer, but she has taken classes and workshops with quite a few since retiring to Boulder eight years ago.

"Sure," she says. She walks to the foot of my gurney, takes my toes in her hands and closes her eyes. She talks me through an exercise that one of her favorite teachers taught her, one in which she directs some of her life force to move down her arms and through her hands into my body, where it moves up from my feet all the way to my head and back again.

"Head ... to toe," she says slowly, her voice like gentle waves. "Head ... to toe." As she speaks, I visualize healing energy moving up and down my broken body, its sparkling light coating every inch of me as it passes through and back again. Normally, my inner smart-aleck would interject a few sarcastic comments, but today, right now, I'm open to whatever healing is available from that which I can neither see nor touch.

A nurse arrives and gives me a dose of Versed to relax me for the biopsy. Mom says goodbye and reassures me that she'll be waiting right here for me. I'm wheeled into a large operating room and I feel small in comparison on the gurney. The doctor explains that I'll be awake for the procedure and that they have to put a lightweight blue drape over my upper body, face included, to keep the area sterile. This is as much detail of the biopsy as he seems willing to share. The drape is made of paper and it doesn't inhibit my breathing, but lying under it, I feel claustrophobic, borderline panicked.

"Please turn your face to the left," says the doctor. I comply and a medical assistant holds my head firmly in place as insurance against any movement.

"Here comes the pinch," he adds, plunging a thin tube into my jugular vein. It hurts like hell despite the medication I was given, but I remain still, stoic even, as tears stream down the left side of my face.

Don't move, don't move, don't move, I repeat silently. *Over soon, over soon, over soon.* My thoughts become mantras that I cling to for survival.

The doctor feeds more of the tubing into the opening in my neck until it reaches the main vein of the liver. After X-rays are taken, he threads a small biopsy needle through the tube. I hear a muffled sound deep within my body. *Click.* It sounds just like the noise when I clip Spike's nails after a bath.

"You just cut a piece of my liver, didn't you?" I ask from under my drape.

"Yes," says the doctor, "but you can't possibly have heard it."

"I did." *Mr. Know-it-all.*

Click.

There it is again. But this time, I keep my observation to myself. *Click. Click. Click.* Three more times I hear the soft sound inside my body.

"All done," says the doctor, pulling the tubing out of my neck and removing the drape. The light of the room momentarily blinds me. The medical assistant cleans the biopsy area and tapes a gauze pad over it. It still hurts more than I imagine it should.

"You took five pieces," I say to the doctor.

He looks surprised. "How would you know that?" he replies with a patronizing air.

"I told you. I heard it. Each and every one."

03/24/00—Around 9 p.m., Jeff called to relay the results of one of the liver tests. Negative. When he seemed perturbed that yet another test had come up with yet another big zero, I laughed and said, "You want a box, don't you—a diagnosis that's neat and tidy." He said no, he just wanted Lauren better. I said, "She's Lauren and she'll do things in her own good time."

13

I'M TIRED AND CRABBY from another sleepless night, but Phil, the alternative healer Mom found through her network of Boulder friends, has arrived for our appointment. Mom greets him at the door and leads him to my bedside. A thin middle-aged man with a peaceful demeanor, he is here to do a "healing" on my chakras and aura, which—he explains—will help heal my "spirit body." I assume a healed spirit body will translate to a healed physical body. At this point, I'm open to anything. My doctors vetoed acupuncture, herbs, and massage, but approved this visit after determining there was no threat to me, nor, I suspect, to their traditional approach to medicine. I imagine them rolling their eyes as they discussed my desire to include alternative healing techniques in my treatment, but I don't care. They've had three weeks to solve this puzzle and they haven't. This is *my* illness and I'm ready to branch out, to expand my realm of possibilities for healing.

Lying quietly on my bed, I try to stay awake as Phil speaks with Mom, who takes notes in the same blue notebook she's carried with her since this ordeal began. Eventually, I give in to exhaustion and close my eyes.

"I'm going to go into a light trance now," he says. "We'll start with a brief prayer for healing and understanding of what is going on." I hear him breathing deeply and slowly, in no apparent rush. After a few minutes of silence, Phil says, "Lauren, can you please say your full name aloud for me?"

"Lauren Ward Larsen," I say, my eyes still closed. I hear him continue to breathe deeply, slowly, rhythmically.

"I'm using the image of a white rose as a symbol for Lauren's spirit," he tells my mother. His voice is soft, yet confident. It lacks the airy-fairy quality I used to use when imitating my concept of a New Age healer, back when I was so smug about things I didn't understand or couldn't easily confirm with my own two eyes.

"There is a white vibration around the rose," continues Phil. "This is healing light that's being directed at her in the form of meditations and prayers from others." The idea that others are thinking of me and helping in whatever spiritual ways they choose comforts me greatly. It reminds me of a scene from *It's a Wonderful Life,* in which friends and neighbors are praying for George Bailey, and when critical mass is achieved, Clarence Oddbody, Angel Second Class, is sent to earth to help. I could use an angel about now. I'm tired of hospital life, the lack of a definitive prognosis, the pain.

"In the center of the rose is a gold color that wants to come out," says Phil. "But it's inhibited for some reason. Lauren's spirit may be out of alignment." He explains that my soul is showing him a pinkish-lavender color, representing optimal health. "This is where she wants to be," he says to Mom. "This bright energy also represents her sharing her healing and love with others, as well as using her intuition more." I have no idea what this means, but I don't feel like asking for clarification.

"I see hard work and struggle associated with Lauren being on her spiritual path," he continues. "I'm seeing her in a past life as a monk, cloistered away from the outside world, which made following her path easy." I open my eyes and look at him, but his eyes are closed. Why is he talking past lives? I just want to feel better *now.* In *this* life.

"Her spirit is ready for healing," says Phil. "But it isn't easy for her spirit to be close to her body right now because of the pain and discomfort the body is experiencing. Her spirit is hovering right over her body and staying close to it, but not in it." As he says this, Phil puts his hands in front of himself as if he's touching something that neither Mom nor I can see. But something in his description of my spirit being outside of my body resonates with me. He has put into words what I've been feeling ever since the encephalopathy subsided ten days ago, the experience of being here, yet not really *being* here.

Phil returns to the subject of gold light, specifically the healing gold light that is within the rose representing my spirit. He sees an impediment keeping the healing gold from emerging—namely, the major life transition brought on by the birth of Clare and the responsibilities that accompany motherhood. I have a fear of this major life change, Phil explains, and therefore asked my spirit to shut down my body for some time as a protective measure; thus the health issues.

Again, I am both intrigued and resistant. The conscious me, the Lauren I have been to the outside world for thirty-eight years now, thinks this is bullshit, that my illness is nothing more than a twist of bad luck in which I'm the unwitting victim. And yet something in Phil's words resonates with me in a way that I am loathe to admit, even to myself. Now agitated, I want him to finish whatever it is he's doing and leave. But I say nothing as I once again close my eyes.

Phil says he's asking one of my spirit guides to replenish the layers of my aura and that different colors are used to do this. He's talking with my spirit, he says, to regenerate the affinity and love I have for myself and others. Next, he moves on to my chakras, the seven energy centers of my spiritual body that he's now clearing. I hear his breathing become more labored. I open my eyes to see him, with eyes closed, moving his hands about as if he is pulling imaginary ropes out of different areas of my body and casting them aside. He begins over the base of my spine—my "survival" chakra, he calls it—and moves to the top of my head to my "crown" chakra.

"I'm being told that her third chakra needs a lot of help," he says, as casually as a mechanic might say I need a new fan belt. Not surprisingly, the third chakra is based in the solar plexus, the area of my liver, kidneys, and the giant blood clot. He re-checks my chakras to make sure there is still a little string, as he calls it, keeping them attached to my physical form. His hands are still in motion above my body, but not once does he actu-ally touch me. I resist the urge to scoff at his seemingly silly pantomimes, yet I sense that the true source of my resistance to Phil's work is his earlier comment that I was afraid of the tran-sition to motherhood. *I wanted this baby, dammit! Why would I be afraid of being a mother?*

"I'm going to work on getting Lauren's kundalini turned on again," Phil says, addressing my mother. He describes kundalini as a powerful energy running from the base of the spine to the head, which can be used as a healing force for the body. He asks me to picture a reservoir holding the kundalini at the base of my spine. When activated, he explains, kundalini rushes up the spine like a whale spout.

"Do you feel more awake, Lauren? Something that feels like more lightness?" Phil asks.

"Yes," I say. Or am I imagining it?

"I'm feeling a shift in her spiritual energy," he says to my mother. "It's integrating more with her body rather than hover-ing above it."

Phil asks me to close my eyes and visualize a gold sphere above my head that is filled with healing energy. He tells me to see it spilling over, coating my body. To draw off any static negative energy, I should visualize a tube running from the base of my spine down into the center of the earth. This "grounding cord" will take away any negative energy that blocks my heal-ing. He instructs me to do this exercise at least once every day. I agree, still not sure what I think about all this.

I keep my eyes closed and hear Phil make a series of gasping sighs, which he tells my mother is his way of clearing my en-

ergy from his body now that his work is done. Then he moves to
her side of the room and sits for the first time in the hour or so
that he's been with us. Despite my earlier agitation with some
of his insights, I feel peaceful. Unconcerned with the formali-
ties of saying goodbye and thank you, I drift off to sleep.

*03/25/00—Phil explained that this illness has changed Lauren's
energy, the aspect of herself as a spirit. Others may not recognize
her as being the same as she was before the illness. Her wellness may
require solitude, not as an escape, but as time for self-healing and in-
trospection. Phil sees her as changing her career direction—looking
within and uncovering a path different from the corporate world.
The physical pain represents the impasse between where she is and
the new life change. When Lauren told him, "I hate the pain," Phil
said he saw it as a way to move forward. It's part of the learning,
the process, the transition to her new life.*

In the early afternoon another visitor knocks at my door—
Amy, who concerns herself only with the physical aspects of my
recovery. There will be no talk of auras or chakras. Amy is holding a clear plastic box about the size of a hardcover book. It has
a blue tube attached at the top of it, the end of which she asks
me to put in my mouth. She coaches me through several deep
breaths, each one pulling the lightweight floor of the plastic box
upward to register the strength of my oxygen intake.

"Try to make the floor of the box float up to the number ten,"
she says, goading me to expand my lung capacity. How hard can
it be? I draw in as much oxygen as I can, until my lungs feel like
they might burst if I force in one more molecule of air. The floor
of the breathing contraption rises up and stops at the number
two. Frustrated, I release the air in my lungs with a gasp, and it
takes me a full minute for my breathing to be steady. Thoughts
of my previous cardiovascular strength taunt me and I will myself not to cry.

"Let's try again," says Amy. Over the next twenty minutes, she coaches me through five more attempts to register a ten on the breathing box. I never make it past three.

Next up is walking. I manage to grab the triangular bar hanging down from a pole over my bed and pull myself up to a sitting position without help. I rest here for several minutes, allowing my equilibrium to return. A nurse slides my slippers onto my feet and places my walker in front of me. I grab the sides of the walker and rise to standing, my energy considerably stronger than it was this morning—a result of Phil's visit? I shuffle eight feet to the commode, shift my grip from the walker to the arms of the commode and lower myself onto it. Within minutes, my body responds. Again, I push myself up to standing, as Mom, Jeff, and two nurses look on, impressed. One of the nurses wipes my bottom as I clutch the walker. I'm feeling invincible, so instead of returning to the hospital bed, I move toward the door. Down the hallway I go, aware that I'm showing off. I pass the little kitchen on the left, make an about-face, and return to my room. My pace is slow, but this is the longest walk I've done while in the hospital, at least twenty-five yards. By the time I make it back to my bed, I have been up for more than half an hour. Amy is pleased. I too am fully aware of what an accomplishment today's physical therapy session has been. Though dizzy, I can feel my strength returning.

My BUN numbers—blood urea nitrogen—are up, indicating the need for another blood cleansing, so the dialysis equipment is once again wheeled into my room. Jeff knows that this is a simple procedure for me, so when Mom encourages him to take some time for himself, he readily agrees. He makes plans to walk Spike with a friend and then meet several other friends for cocktails.

When the dialysis procedure is over, I decide to use the commode before dinner arrives. This time, I need the help of two nurses to get there. Given my stellar performance earlier in the day, no one is disappointed, myself included. Once settled on the commode, the nurses leave me in Mom's care. A few minutes pass when suddenly I feel my head tilt backward as if my neck has turned to rubber. I'm unable to see anything except the color of gold. I hear Mom's voice saying my name, but am unable to form the words to tell her that I'm fine. I try gesturing with my hands, but I can't move them either.

"Lauren, are you okay?" Her voice is louder than usual and has an edge of frenzied concern.

I'm fine, really I'm fine, I try to say, but I can't get the words out of my mouth.

"Lauren!" she shouts.

I'm right here! I try to yell back. But I'm frozen in this state of paralysis, fully aware that I'm unable to communicate, aware that it must seem as if I'm in trouble and yet, oddly, feeling perfectly fine.

"Nurse!" she yells. "I need help! STAT!"

Stat? Where the hell did she learn the term "stat"?

"NURSE!" she yells again.

Mom! I'm right here!

And yet I'm not. I remain in this strange place of blinding gold light where I can neither move nor speak.

"Lauren!" I hear right in front of my face. It's one of my regular nurses. "Lauren!" she repeats again and again.

I try so hard to answer her, but I still can't get the words out. Time passes—two minutes? Three? I blink my eyes and suddenly I can see again. Mom looks both scared and relieved. I tell her I'm okay and this time I hear the words leave my mouth. There are others in the room now—several nurses and nurses' aides. I'm embarrassed for causing such a commotion.

"Lauren, how do you feel?" asks one of the nurses.

"Dizzy," I say. "Dizzy and weak."

"Blood pressure's seventy-eight over forty," says another nurse, as she unwraps a blood pressure cuff from my right arm.

Several people pull me to standing and move me to my bed, where I lie back and close my eyes to rest. Well, *that* was interesting, I think. Things settle down and one by one, the hospital staff leaves my room until I'm alone with Mom.

"Know where I was?" I ask.

"No. Where?" she replies.

"I was in the gold."

14

I AM HUNCHED OVER IN THE PADDED CHAIR across from my hospital bed. Two pillows tucked under me ease the discomfort, but I loathe the daily ritual of being hauled out of bed and propped up in this chair, this god-awful ugly chair. I feel nauseous and afraid, fearful of throwing up all those calories from breakfast that I had such a hard time swallowing: the three bites of scrambled egg, the half-slice of rubbery toast, the cup of juice. If I puke, I have to begin counting all over again. Why do they nag me so much about eating? I'm not hungry. Nothing sounds good. Nothing tastes good. How can it when my mouth and throat are coated in thrush? I close my eyes and hope the swaying and spinning will pass.

And now *he* is here. Ichabod—not his real name, but it's what I call him. Not to his face. Just to myself. And to my husband. And my family. And maybe to some of the nurses, like Carol and Susan, whose kindness is so sincerely offered I often want to cry with relief in their presence. My personal support team— and especially Jeff—universally dislikes Ichabod. Tall and lean, with a pinched face, he managed to alienate my husband and family during the first few days of my hospitalization by prefacing almost every medical opinion he rendered with the phrase "Well, if she lives …".

Morning rounds are in progress and Ichabod is standing in front of my chair, a gaggle of interns and residents surrounding him. I avoid looking directly into his eyes.

"Lauren?" he says. I ignore him.

He tells me I'm still not eating enough, that I need to consume at least 2,400 calories a day. I barely got 200 down at breakfast. Ichabod says another feeding tube will be inserted tomorrow morning if I don't prove that I can eat more today. I find his demeanor a bit too smug, his voice unnecessarily loud, as if I'm retarded or deaf or both. I hate him, and I want him to go away.

"Lauren? Do you think you can try to eat more for me today?" he says.

For you? For you I'll do nothing!

I want to tell Ichabod to shove his stethoscope up his ass. I want to tell him I've had enough of his condescending attitude. But I say nothing, give no sign of the strong-willed smart-ass I used to be. The old me, the non-sick me, would have responded with the perfect degree of contempt disguised as a clever quip, like a timed-release sarcasm pill, the full effect of which would not be felt until after he'd left my room. Instead I avert my eyes, bow my head, and remain mute, all the while silently willing Ichabod to disappear.

Go away. Go away. Just go away.

03/26/00—Jeff again stayed overnight at the hospital. Neither he nor Lauren slept for shit.

Mom arrives shortly after morning rounds and finds me still sitting in the chair, despondent. Jeff leaves to get another latte, his lack of sleep apparent from his blank expression.

"What's up?" she asks.

"My recovery is taking so long," I say. "I'm tired and depressed and I hurt. And I want to get back in bed, but I don't think my legs are going to hold me when I stand up." I feel my face crumple in that way it does preceding a good cry. Mom hands me a tissue, but as I take it I realize my eyes are still dry.

"I don't even have any tears," I say, my face continuing to scrunch up like an amateur actor's portrayal of sorrow. The inability to perform the simplest of tasks—in this case weeping—further fuels my despondency.

"Try to keep focusing on the big picture, Lauren," Mom says. "Think of how far you've come since this began."

I try, but it doesn't help.

At lunchtime, I'm obsessed with proving I can eat enough to satisfy the doctors, but nothing on the tray looks appealing and no amount of encouragement from Mom gets the food to go down. Despite the knowledge that another nasogastric tube lies in my future, I push the lunch tray away, the majority of its contents left untouched.

Jeff leaves the hospital to shower, walk Spike, and bring her to the hospital for a visit. Having explained my close connection with my dog to my doctors and assuring them of Spike's vast experience visiting hospitals through our SPCA pet-therapy work, Jeff persuaded them to ignore the rules and allow a dog in the Transitional ICU. But only on a Sunday, they'd cautioned. Today is Sunday.

When Spike arrives, she doesn't pull on her leash as is typical. She stays close to Jeff's leg, looking nervous, her tail down. Glancing around the room, she looks right at me, but registers nothing in the way of recognition. We haven't seen each other for nearly a month and I must look odd to her. And smell funny. My body has become so sensitive that even a sponge bath has been out of the question since my arrival. I'm still deep yellow from the jaundice, my skin greasy from its attempts to eliminate toxins through my pores. Jeff sets a small bag of dog treats on the bed next to my left hand. I pull one out and hold it in Spike's direction.

"Here, Spikey," I say. She strains forward with her head, her paws firmly in place as if she's standing on a cliff, careful not to get too close to the edge. Gently, she pulls the biscuit from my hand, retreats, and chews it. I could be a complete stranger, just another sick person she's met in her three years of visiting hospital patients, me tucking treats into their feeble hands to initiate the animal-human interaction. The only difference is that Spike's tail is usually wagging during these visits. But today, right now, her tail remains between her legs.

I feed Spike a few more treats, pretending that her indifference doesn't bother me, and soon I mimic her lack of interest, turn and stare out the window at the midday San Francisco fog. Jeff guides Spike to a chair across the room and sits down. She lies on the floor beside him, resting her head on her front paws. To the hospital personnel, Spike is the picture of calm. But I know better. She's frightened, tense, and wants one thing: to flee, to get away—posthaste—from the big yellow monster that looks vaguely like her mother.

03/26/00—We think Spike is having a problem with abandonment issues, which is understandable. But when she ignored Lauren, it only added to Lauren's depression.

Late that afternoon, Pam arrives, her arms loaded with grocery and party-store bags. Earlier today, when she offered to bring in food and drink so we could all watch the Academy Awards together, Jeff and Mom readily agreed. Anything to improve the mood of week four in the hospital.

"Can't have an Oscar party without the right decorations," she says, pulling supplies from one of the bags. She moves about the room, hanging Hollywood-motif decorations: big gold stars; cardboard cutouts of director's chairs, megaphones, and movie cameras; and gold metallic garland, which she wraps around the pole over my bed. Mom makes comments meant to establish a festive mood. *You really outdid yourself, Pam! This'll be some party!*

I recognize that they're trying hard to create a distraction, perhaps for themselves as much as for me, but it all feels forced, borderline patronizing, and I swallow my resentment like a pill. None of us, including me, seems willing to acknowledge the elephant in the room—the big depressed elephant who's getting neither better nor worse, who wants only to lash out at everyone, regardless of how kind they've been or how much time they've dedicated to helping me.

From my hospital bed, I feign interest in the activity around me, intermittently sucking on the straw of my fourth container of Resource. Each eight-ounce carton equals one-fifth of the daily calories required to avoid having another feeding tube inserted, and I've already calculated that if I drink five Resources each day, I won't have to eat any solid food. The thrush makes food taste awful and swallowing difficult, so I continue forcing down the chalky-tasting fluid.

Pam pulls something else from her bags and holds it up for Mom to see. Both women laugh. "I couldn't resist," says Pam. She walks to the foot of my bed and proudly displays a novelty store plaque with a big plastic fish on it. The caption reads: *Best Fishes*. I offer a perfunctory smile.

"Wait! Here's the best part," says Pam. She pushes a little red button on the plaque and the plastic fish comes to life, its head and tail flipping mechanically outward, its mouth opening and closing as it sings, "Don't worry, be happy." Mom and Pam laugh even harder.

How annoying.

Offering an insincere chuckle, I try hard not to be a wet blanket on their amusement. Wracked with guilt that they've all put their own lives on hold to help me, I play along with these attempts to make me happy rather than express what I'm truly feeling—the deepest sort of loneliness that comes from knowing that the people around me, those who hold me dearest, can't even begin to understand the physical and emotional hell that I've been living since Clare's birth. Not one.

Jeff returns from taking Spike home, and as he walks into the room, Mom tells him to look at the plaque, now hanging on the wall in place of a bland floral print. He gives a snicker—forced, like mine was.

"Push the button," she says. He does, and again laughs insincerely. Even a chorus of a thousand singing fish wouldn't improve our situation.

Pam turns on the television in the corner of the room, keeps the volume low, and scans the channels until she finds the Oscars. Beautiful celebrities in expensive designer gowns and tuxedos make their way down the packed red carpet toward the Shrine Auditorium.

"What have you got there?" asks Jeff, indicating the two grocery bags. Pam begins unloading carton after carton of prepared foods: pasta salads, cheeses, and a variety of hors d'oeuvres and desserts, all foods Pam knows I'd love under normal circumstances, all specially selected to coax me into eating something—*anything*—to boost my caloric intake. Yet nothing tempts me. Instead, I feel repulsed as I scan the makeshift buffet that's being set up on my bedside table. Jeff *oohs* and *ahhs* at all the choices, his tone now sincere, and begins filling a Hollywood-themed paper plate with food.

As I continue to feign interest, I feel something stir in my gut. Before I can utter a word of warning, the entire contents of my stomach—all four cartons of Resource—come spewing from my mouth. Puke covers my hospital gown, the bed, even part of the table on which the Oscar party buffet is arranged. The involuntary convulsions of my stomach continue, and Mom hands me a small trash can. I'm tempted to laugh at the futility of the gesture, but instead I cry. I've lost all those hard-earned calories in one fit of projectile vomiting. My greatest fear at this moment is that a doctor will appear any minute, feeding-tube kit in hand.

Jeff rubs my back, tries to comfort me. Pam turns the television off. A nurse moves around my bed, carefully and efficiently replacing the soiled linens with clean ones. Mom gathers the containers of food, tossing the ones that were in the line of fire into a separate bag to be thrown away. The party is over. And after Pam leaves, I insist that the fish plaque be taken off the wall and sent to the children's ward. I never want to see it again.

03/26/00—Lauren told us she feels like she has no control in her life. She doesn't want anyone bringing food in for her or doing things for her, no matter how thoughtful they're trying to be. She doesn't want anyone to stay overnight. She wants to direct who does what. This is the only way she can exercise some control.

The following morning, Karen phones from Pennsylvania to coach me through the process of getting another feeding tube inserted, offering tips on how to make it go more smoothly. I melt into tears and ask about other options, such as a feeding tube inserted directly into my belly, anything to avoid the constant ache of a tube lodged in my nasal passages. Patiently, she explains why a nasogastric tube is the best approach. Nothing she says differs from what my doctors have been telling me, but hearing it from her makes it more believable. Accepting that I have no other options, I sob even more. It sounds as if she too is crying on the other end of the telephone.

"Lauren, you know we all love you so much that any of us would take your place if we could," Karen says. She pauses. "In fact, if the docs ask, I'll volunteer Tim." We both laugh, our love of immature humor overriding our mutual sadness. When I hang up the phone, an intern arrives with a feeding-tube kit and once again, I begin receiving nutrition through my nose.

15

MOM WALKS BESIDE THE GURNEY as I'm wheeled to the magnetic imaging department for an abdominal MRI. My doctors are concerned that the giant clot still resting on top of my uterus is causing infection. The MRI technician greets our gurney, hands my mother a clipboard of paperwork for her signature, and turns to me. He's young, maybe early thirties, and his voice is reassuring, not rushed. Two other patients in wheelchairs await his services outside the door, but the severity of my case trumped their place in line. He hands me a paper cup of fluid and explains that drinking this dye will help with the imaging process. He apologizes in advance for its taste, and with Mom holding my shoulders up, I drain the cup. Then he says something about an enema.

"Enema?" I repeat. I've never had an enema and I find the thought disturbing, more so when he tells me I'll be "holding it" for the duration of the MRI process.

"Don't worry," he says, showing me a tube with a special cap on one end. "Once we insert this little balloon-like tip in your rectum, we'll inflate it. It'll be impossible for the enema to leak out, so you won't need to do a thing."

"Good, because I don't have any control down there," I say.

"Not a problem," he says.

Two orderlies transfer my body to the padded table connected to the MRI machine. It's about the size of a VW bug and there's a large opening at the foot of the table, giving the appearance of a tunnel. The technician asks me to bend my legs at the knees so he can insert the enema tube.

"She can't do that," Mom tells him.

"Not a problem," he says again. He and Mom each take a leg and bend it for me, holding my feet in place so they don't slide down the length of the table. Mom holds both legs while the technician guides the enema tube into position and turns a faucet handle on another machine, starting the flow of water into my colon. He turns the water off, presses a different button, and now I feel a slight sensation at the base of my spine as the end of the enema tube inflates.

"It feels weird, like I'm going to poop any minute," I say. "You sure this thing will hold?"

"Positive," he says.

"Has anyone ever blown out the enema while lying in the MRI machine?"

"Never."

"Because that looks like a pretty expensive piece of equipment you've got there."

"It is."

His smile tells me he's amused by my concern. Taking my legs from Mom, he lowers them to the table and pushes a button on the side of the machine. I feel myself moving toward the tunnel, feet first. When all but my head is inside, the table stops moving and he asks Mom to follow him into the small viewing room about ten feet from the massive machine. I hear his voice over the intercom, and with a quick glance to the left I see him and Mom behind a picture window.

"Okay, Lauren, you're doing great so far," he says, his voice somewhat tinny from the distortion of the audio system. "Now I need you to lie very still for about thirty minutes while we get these images. It's pretty loud, okay? Try to hang in there, but if you absolutely need me to stop the machine, you can say so. I'll be able to hear you over the noise. Ready?"

"Ready," I say.

The room is flooded with the cacophonous thumping of the MRI machine as it creates a visual road map of my guts. The noise doesn't bother me, but the sensation that I'm about to lose control of my bowels does. He said it's impossible to blow out the enema, I tell myself. He said I didn't need to try to hold it, so I don't. I assume the sensation of pooping is simply what it feels like to have an enema balloon in my rectum. Half an hour later the machine is shut off and I open my eyes to see the technician standing over me.

"How was that?" he asks.

"I think I blew out the enema," I say.

"Not possible."

"Better check."

He pushes a button and peers into the machine as my body makes its slow migration out of the tunnel. He looks surprised, regains his facial composure, and turns back to me.

"Yep," he says. "You blew out the enema."

"Sorry," I say, offering a weak smile of apology.

03/27/00—Jeff told Lauren he was running out to buy some dinner to eat with her—and did she want anything. "Yes, a milkshake." How about a hamburger? "Yes." Onion rings? "Yes." Off he went. Alas, the guy at the restaurant forgot to put the shakes in the bag. Jeff walked back up the hill and discovered the error in Lauren's room. He suggested to Lauren that they eat their burgers and onion rings first, and then he'd go back for the shakes. Lauren said sharply, "Honnnnn!" So Jeff went back down the hill for the shakes, and predictably, by the time he returned Lauren was asleep. Ah well ...

Bob stops by during evening rounds to discuss the results of the abdominal MRI. My liver has doubled in size since it failed after Clare's delivery.

"It's a textbook regeneration," he says to me, Jeff, and Mom. I bet it feels good for him to finally be able to share good news with us.

My uterus, however, is still quite large—the size it would be if I were four months pregnant, he explains. More tests are needed, so the following morning I'm again wheeled down to the imaging department. This time, a transvaginal ultrasound will be performed to make sure there are no blood clots inside my uterus. Again, Mom remains at my side. I'm taken to a different area of the imaging wing where we meet the ultrasound technician, who explains the procedure using words like *insertion* and *vagina*, while holding what appears to be a white billy club. This *probe*, as he calls it, will take internal images while inside my vagina. I can remain as I am, prone on the gurney. I just need to bend my legs at the knees, he explains. Mom and I share a quick glance.

"She can't," says Mom, for the second time in the past twenty-four hours.

The technician helps my mother position my legs properly, spreading them apart as he does so. When he lets go, one of my legs flops off to the side and he quickly grabs it. He and Mom struggle to find a way to keep my legs bent and spread while also preventing my feet from sliding out from under them. He suggests that they move the gurney against a wall, so he can prop up one of my legs. He'll hold the other one while maneuvering the probe, and Mom will push down on the tops of my feet, so my legs won't slide off the gurney pad. All three of us seem to find the humor in the situation, and as Mom moves into position at my feet, I can't help but giggle at her direct view of my undraped vagina.

"Is this more of me than you'd hoped to be seeing?" I ask her.

The technician slides the probe inside my body and I stop laughing. The doctors estimate that the blood clot resting on top of my uterus is the size of a basketball, and pockets of air and fluid continue to form in my abdomen on a daily basis. Now the pressure of the probe—one more thing vying for space in there—takes my breath away. I grimace, sucking in air through gritted teeth.

"You okay?" Mom asks.

"Yeah," I say, a complete lie.

"Sorry about this," says the technician. "I'll try to be quick." A few minutes pass in silence as he continues securing ultrasound images from different angles inside my vagina.

"This is the only sex I've had in months," I say, before wincing at another stab of pain.

Maybe laughter *isn't* the best medicine. But if I can still crack a joke, perhaps I can make it through another procedure, another day.

16

Sabra rubs lavender lotion on my hands as I rest following another three-hour dialysis session. Lavender is my favorite aromatherapy scent, but right now I feel like I may vomit at what I can only describe as its stench. I yank my bony hand from her gentle grip.

"Sorry," I say. I try explaining my heightened sense of smell to Sabra, Mom, and Jeff, but their faces tell me they don't understand how lavender could smell rancid. I don't understand either, but it does. So does the smell of the saline solution whenever my IV line is flushed to keep it from developing bacteria. "But saline solution doesn't have a smell," said one of my nurses the other day. *You're clueless*, I thought, turning my head away and covering my nose with the blankets so I wouldn't vomit. And now, with the scent of lavender offending my senses, I'm again reminded that my nurses, doctors, family, and friends can travel this road only so far with me. The full extent of the journey will never be experienced by anyone but me. And right now, what I'm experiencing is nausea.

"I understand," Sabra says, obviously lying.

Sabra and I met four years ago when I relocated to San Francisco and she worked as an editor for my new employer. Fast friends from the start, we were both unwilling to succumb to the rampant cynicism of the publishing world. With tongues firmly imbedded in cheeks, we secretly called ourselves The Rainbow Girls. Anytime either of us felt beaten down by the negativity of a coworker or the verbal abuse of an irate author, we'd hustle to the other's office, shut the door, and proclaim that we were "in serious need of a rainbow." The other would immediately move her hands in an exaggerated arc overhead, as if making an imaginary rainbow in the sky. Then we'd laugh ourselves silly as we mocked the source of our agitation until our equilibrium and spirits returned. It worked every time. It's clear to me that Sabra has tried her best to maintain a "rainbow attitude" over the past four weeks. She's been the bearer of all news—both good and bad—to former colleagues, answering questions, gently discouraging those who wanted to drop in unannounced, and helping the human resources department launch the company's inaugural blood drive.

In time, I'll learn about the breakdown she and Pam shared while I was comatose, when Sabra observed that it "felt like death" in my ICU room. I'll learn how she left the hospital two weeks ago uncertain if she would see her rainbow gal-pal alive again, and when she walked into her home and told her husband that she needed a hug, he had none to give, so she slid to the floor and balled herself up tight and small. I'll learn, as will she, that within a year, her marriage will end. But for now, the Sabra who visits me almost daily shares none of her sadness or fears. Instead, she goes out of her way to bring me treats, things she knows the old me would love, such as the gnocchi in Gorgonzola cream sauce she brought from my favorite restaurant, which failed to elicit the desired response. A fierce optimist, Sabra has maintained a steadfast commitment to encouraging me despite my lackluster response to her efforts. But lately I've noticed a slight shift in her demeanor, a crack in that effervescent exterior. Sabra's rainbow is fading. And I'm glad.

The upbeat façade and forced cheerfulness that she—or anyone else, for that matter—delivers to my hospital room agitates me—pisses me off, in fact. Intellectually, I understand that she's trying to give me the rainbow I so badly need, the rainbow that the old Lauren, the one who had never acknowledged the depth of suffering that is possible in life, would've accepted in a heartbeat. But this Lauren—me, here, now—doesn't give a rat's ass about rainbows or optimism or cheerfulness. I'm angry. And I want to stay in my anger.

Mom senses the distance I'm putting between Sabra and me, even asks about it after my friend leaves. I brush off her questions and pretend I don't understand where she got that idea. Later, another alternative healer Mom found through her contacts in Boulder arrives—a reflexologist named Roberta. She begins by taking one of my hands in hers and lightly stroking it, then applying pressure to certain points that correspond with various internal organs. I wonder, as she gently squeezes the fleshy part of my palm, if that's my liver point, and if so, what my liver might be telling her. She moves on to my legs, first rubbing my lower legs in long slow stroking motions. Watching from her chair by the window, Mom's facial expression shifts to one of concern.

"The doctors were worried about the possibility of loosening clots with any form of massage," she says.

"I'm aware of the problems," Roberta says, not unkindly. "These are very superficial strokes, not deep at all." Relaxing, Mom returns to her book.

"I'd like to work on your feet now, Lauren," Roberta says. "Is it okay if I remove your socks?" For my entire stay in the hospital, I've been wearing the same pair of thick hiking socks. There has been no move by anyone to change them, as hygiene has been low on the list of priorities. I nod my consent and she begins to slowly, carefully slip them off.

As the fabric of the socks falls away, so too does the fabric of my feet. Quarter-size pieces of skin hang off each foot, beckoning Roberta to give them that last little tug. My size ten feet—the same ones that were strong enough to carry me across the finish line of six marathons, that carried me to the top of Half Dome in Yosemite during my honeymoon—are now withered and bony. They look like chicken feet, all prickly and meatless.

"Wow," I say. "Kinda gross, huh?"

Roberta begins to rub, then lightly squeeze, the soles of my feet, and I relax into the comfort of her hands. Unlike my earlier response to Sabra's attempt at massaging my limbs, I have no compulsion to withdraw from Roberta's touch. Perhaps it's because of what she is—a professional healer. Or perhaps it's because of what she is not—someone like Sabra, someone I care for so deeply that nothing she does is good enough.

03/29/00—Lauren's clotting time is still down. Her platelets are not working well. Bleeding continues to be her #1 complication. There's still no further progress.

A psychiatric intern stands at the foot of my hospital bed. She is young—late twenties, early thirties perhaps—and pretty, with shoulder-length dark brown hair. She wears a white lab coat and clutches a clipboard like a nervous child clinging to her favorite stuffed animal. I know she's here to evaluate me, to prescribe antidepressants, which my intensive care doctors assured me will help. Too many nights I've lain awake agitated, twitchy, and unable to sleep, and it's wearing on me.

Before this ordeal began I never had trouble sleeping, never took a sleeping pill or antidepressant, didn't even keep a regular supply of ibuprofen in my medicine cabinet. I smugly told others that pharmaceuticals weren't my thing, that I'd rather tough it out, preferring to massage the reflexology points between my thumb and forefinger to ease a headache rather than simply popping a couple of Tylenol. But now—one seizure, two liver biopsies, three weeks of kidney dialysis, and one hundred and eighty pints of blood after my emergency cesarean section—I want to take whatever she'll give me, anything that offers sleep.

Mom sits in the corner of the room by the large window, the book she was reading now face down on her lap. The intern asks a few simple questions, making small talk. Her mannerisms are

stiff, as if she recently read a medical article about the importance of establishing rapport with patients and she is attempt-
ing to put into practice what she learned. I haven't slept more
than an hour at a time for days. *Just give me the damn drugs.*
Her tone shifts, and she no longer maintains eye contact.
"Have you ever considered suicide?" she asks.

The question hangs in the air between us. I steal a look at
my mother, whose raised eyebrows and slightly agape mouth
communicate her thoughts in no uncertain terms. I can almost
hear her saying, *She didn't really ask that, did she?* I'm a month
into this postpartum nightmare with no clear prognosis, while
my baby girl is living four hundred miles away because neither
my husband nor I can care for her, and this shrink-in-training
is asking me if I've ever considered suicide? My first instinct is
to lash out with caustic sarcasm. *Me? Suicide? Are you kidding?
I'm having the time of my fucking life!*

But I say nothing. Instead I try to figure out what the *right*
answer is. Will being suicidal get me the drugs to sleep? Will
not being suicidal allow me to go home sooner? Regardless, it's
a stupid question.

Must I explain to her how much pain I've been in for a month
now, how frustrating it is to be surrounded by experts who can't
seem to fix me and loved ones whose kindness only annoys me?
Do I tell her how much guilt I feel that my husband, three best
friends, and family members have put their own lives on hold
to be with me, flying in from five different states and taking
shifts with me so I'm never alone? Do I tell her how I lie awake
during the quiet hours of the night wondering what I must've
done to create this massive failure of my body during an event
thousands of women go through daily without incident?

Do I admit that I vacillate between feeling like I've failed my
baby and resenting her very existence? So far, I've only admit-
ted the former. The latter feels too despicable an emotion to
acknowledge to anyone, let alone to myself. Yes, the pregnancy

was unplanned. But I wanted her, truly wanted her, all the more when my husband's fear and emotional distancing at the pregnancy test results threatened to force a choice. I would have chosen her. *I would have!*

But that was then and this is now.

Do I tell this Freud wannabe that I would've terminated the pregnancy without a second thought if I'd known this would happen? That at times I've been consumed with ending the excruciating pain even if it means death? Not suicide, but death.

"No," I say. "I've never considered suicide."

My mother interrupts the psychiatric evaluation and asks the young doctor to leave, citing my need to rest. After she's gone, Mom tells me she's going to find the head of the ICU and tell him she doesn't want "that woman" involved in my care or interacting with me anymore.

Later that afternoon, the hospital's head psychiatrist comes to my room and asks me a few questions. How long have I been unable to sleep through the night? What's the longest I've slept in one stretch over the past week? Am I feeling anxious or agitated because of this? Yes? Okay, let's get you something that will help, he tells me. Small doses of antidepressant and antianxiety medications should do the trick. He never mentions the word *suicide*.

Hours later, two new prescriptions are added to my regimen. I take the pills and drift off almost immediately. I do not awaken when I inadvertently pull the feeding tube from my nose. I do not awaken when I'm transfused with two more bags of blood. I do not awaken for a full five hours.

Tonight, I have been given the blessed gift of sleep.

17

THOUGH THE LATEST FEEDING TUBE remains firmly taped to my face, the nutritional formula that ran through it, and consequently through my body at warp speed, has been discontinued. Multiple diarrhea attacks caused a sleepless night and several sheet changes because I couldn't get to the bedpan in time. And unlike the experience of lying in my own feces during my crazy phase, there is no joy or satisfaction now that my thinking is more lucid. Now, shitting myself is just one more reminder that I'm not in control of my body and, therefore, not in control of my life. Shit and control go hand in hand, I'm learning. Crying, I call Jeff at five in the morning and ask him to come back to the hospital.

When Mom arrives a few hours later, she attempts to cheer me up with details of who's coming to town next. At this point in my care, my family members have been taking breaks to return to their homes in Pennsylvania, Kentucky, Michigan, southern California, and Colorado, understanding that their well-being is an imperative ingredient for survival, theirs as well as mine.

"John's flight lands at 11:50 this morning," Mom says, reading from her blue notebook. I offer no response as I lie still, eyes closed, exhausted from the scatological crisis of last night.

"And Karen gets in around the same time tomorrow," she adds. Again I say nothing. Mom laughs and says, "I'm sure you don't give a shit."

I open my eyes and look at my mother. "No," I say, "I give *too much* shit."

Michael believes the feeding formula I was given is too rich for my system, so he and the ICU dietician arrive to review my chart and discuss different options. There is talk of high blood counts, infection, and another surgery—possibly being performed as soon as tomorrow morning. I have overheard much discussion about this additional surgery for several days now. Some of the experts are hopeful that it will allow them to clean up my organs, remove the giant blood clot, and see what else might be going on that has escaped detection by the myriad tests performed to date. Some fear it may disrupt the delicate balance of my gut right now. Some mention the possibility of a complete hysterectomy.

As bizarre as it seems, I'm in favor of another surgery because I see it as forward movement, one way or another, and I make my amateur opinion known to anyone who will listen. *Just take it all—the blood clot, the uterus, and whatever the hell else you want.* I'm sick of being sick. And I want to go home.

"It seems like everything the doctors are doing to my body is screwing me up more," I complain to Mom when we're alone. "I want to go home and do alternative approaches."

"I want you to do that, too, Lauren," Mom says. "But your body is still very sick," she adds. "You really need western medicine right now. And remember, we *are* doing some alternative treatments." Satisfied with her response, I again close my eyes to rest. Sometimes, a simple acknowledgment of my frustration is all I need.

That afternoon, the latest in our lineup of alternative healers arrives. Dusa is short, tiny in fact, with one thick braid running down her back all the way to her tailbone. My thinking is somewhat foggy again. She appears to be a thirty-something African-American, when in reality she is of Indian descent and pushing sixty. She's wearing my favorite color, purple, and she has a small diamond stud in her nose.

Her thick Brooklyn accent becomes apparent as she and Mom make their introductions and share pretreatment pleasantries. She sets up her bag as if she's a country doctor on a house call. With her supplies arranged, Dusa turns her attention to me. Mom moves to her usual chair, and my stepdad, who arrived several hours ago, remains seated by the window. I'm aware of John's skepticism of all things alternative, let alone anything that hints at being spiritually oriented, but right now that doesn't concern me. In Dusa's presence I feel comfort, and I intend to enjoy this feeling while it lasts. *I like this one,* I think, as I close my eyes and open to the possibilities.

Dusa begins by asking my permission to place various small stones on different parts of my body. I am momentarily taken aback. Someone *asked* my permission to do something to me.

"Sure," I say. Then I watch as she delicately places a purple amethyst on one of my legs, a reddish-white crystal on the other, and more crystals of varying color and shape on my shoulders, abdomen, and chest. She doesn't explain why she's doing this and I don't ask. I'm content to simply receive whatever it is she has to offer. All the rocks in place, I close my eyes and relax. Minutes pass and I realize Dusa hasn't yet touched me. I open my eyes—just a crack—and see that she is moving her hands up and down the length of my body, about five inches above it, and she appears to be smoothing down an imaginary outer shell. She doesn't seem at all self-conscious about this odd pantomime of hers, as if it were as natural to my care as giving me another injection or hanging another bag of blood. I give way to the calm that saturates my body and close my eyes. Ten, maybe fifteen minutes pass. Dusa touches my shoulder the way you would gently wake someone from a nap on an airplane before landing.

"Do you have anything to say?" she asks. Her voice is rich and maternal, nurturing in ways I never imagined a Brooklyn accent could be.

"I'm tired of this place," I whisper.

"I see this as a spiritual challenge for you," she says.

From her corner, Mom makes a joke about wanting Dusa to perform a one-shot miracle, and both my mother and I laugh. "*Lauren* will do that," Dusa says to Mom. "She'll heal herself." Her voice is calm and confident, and I believe her. I do. "The body has its own pharmacy," she adds. "And one way to access it is through laughter."

She resumes the smoothing motions of her hands over my body, and it looks as though she's pushing something from the area over my heart downward to cover my midsection, like stretching out pizza dough. I feel something release from deep within my abdomen. An hour passes, Dusa moving her hands above every inch of my body, me relaxing, feeling better than I have in a long time.

"Is there any place you'd like me to touch you, Lauren?" she asks, waiting patiently while I consider her question.

"My abdomen, please." I have no idea why I want her to put her hands on my swollen and hypersensitive belly, but as they gently rest there, my entire body tingles and I feel good. *Really* good. This time, I'm certain I'm not imagining it.

Dusa begins to pack up her stones, placing each inside a small silk bag with a drawstring. She stops, pulls one back out of the bag and turns to me. "This is for you," she says, handing me a three-inch-long clear crystal that she had placed over my heart during the treatment.

"Thank you," I say, the words unable to express the depth of gratitude I feel.

This crystal will become a symbol of healing for me and will hold a special place of honor on my meditation altar at home. In three years, when Spike is diagnosed with terminal bladder cancer and given a prognosis of "a matter of weeks" from two different veterinary practices, I will hang this crystal in a tiny drawstring bag from her collar, telling my husband, "Hey, it worked for me." And Spike will live for two more years.

All packed up, Dusa says to Mom, "It's important for Lauren's family and friends to touch her, even as she sleeps." Then she turns to me. "Would you like me to call you before your surgery tomorrow morning?" she asks.

"Yes," I reply. And I mean it. I want more Dusa. I don't quite understand it, but I want more of the calm certainty about my imminent wellness that she has given me in our ninety minutes together. Before leaving, she promises to call.

I close my eyes, and soon I feel Mom gently stroking my right arm and hand. It feels good, and I can tell I'm smiling. John, still in the room, has been quietly watching this whole time. Since I've known him, since he and Mom started seeing one another and then married during my sophomore year in college, he has always been reserved when it came to showing emotion, as if any affection that didn't involve his wife was awkward for him. I open my eyes and look at him sitting, hands folded in his lap, in the corner.

"Come on, John," I say. "Grab some skin." And he does.

As my parents rub my arms, I think about the surgery, confirmed for early tomorrow morning, April Fool's Day. How appropriate, I thought when they told me.

Several surgeons are scheduled: Bob, the liver expert who is also my family's favorite doctor; the kidney specialist; my obstetrician; and someone new to my team, an obstetric surgeon whom my family refers to as Keyser Söze. *He's a man of few words*, the head of the ICU told Mom and Jeff, who promptly nicknamed the surgeon after the laconic character in the movie *The Usual Suspects*.

The surgical team has cautioned us against getting our hopes too high. *Just exploratory*, they've said repeatedly. *No guarantees. We won't know anything until we go in.* Despite their call for prudence and realistic expectations, my earlier nonchalance about this surgery is gone, replaced with a calm certainty.

This is it. The turning point.

That evening, I'm startled from a nap by the phone, which was plugged in at my request in case Dusa called. Scanning the room, I see that I'm alone, so I answer the phone myself for the first time since being hospitalized.

"Sluggo!" booms the familiar voice of my friend John. This nickname, which we share, originated during our time working long hours together in New York in the late eighties. If either of us left work before, say, ten o'clock at night, the other would accuse the departing one of being a lazy slug. Over twelve years and three different mutual workplaces, the nickname stuck. Normally, I'm buoyed when I hear this familiar greeting, but tonight I'm disappointed. It's not Dusa.

"Slug, you there?" he says.

"I'm here," I say.

"I'm on my way to the city and I want to come see you." The casualness of John's voice bothers me.

"Please don't," I say.

"Come on, Slug! I'm only ten minutes from the hospital. I won't stay long."

I realize that I'm feeling the same way I've felt every time something painful was done to me in the hospital, every time someone told me it wouldn't hurt, just a small pinch, one more needle, and before I can answer their rhetorical question about whether or not I'm ready, they plow ahead and hurt me anyway, and damn it, I'm sick of it! I want someone to listen! I want to be heard!

"Don't come," I say. And as I hear John begin to protest, I place the handset of the phone back in its cradle.

This is *my* illness. And *I'll* decide who visits.

18

I HEAR THE SOUND OF WAVES crashing on the shoreline, receding, crashing again. I see a kite flying high above as three-year-old Clare giggles and Jeff jogs across the grassy expanse of a park, kite string taut behind him. The scene shifts, and Jeff is now making blueberry pancakes in animal shapes while I read a book to Clare at the kitchen counter. These are my visualizations, the movies I play over and over in my mind as I listen to the surf CD I use to relax. I feel an emotion I haven't felt during my entire month in the hospital—excitement. Not about the kite or the pancakes or even Clare, now a happy toddler in my imagination. The source of my excitement is the surgery that will take place in less than an hour. The shift that I felt during and after Dusa's visit last night has not waned, but strengthened. Today, there will be a miracle. I know it. I feel it.

I look at my right palm, where the crystal from Dusa is held firmly in place by white first-aid tape. One of the nurses suggested we secure it so it wouldn't fall from my hand during the surgery. She understood my need to cling to this talisman, has probably taped many objects of comfort—crosses, rosaries, wedding bands, lockets—to the hands of her surgical patients.

There is activity outside my hospital room and a nurse pokes her head in. "Fifteen minutes, Lauren," she says. Soon I'll be wheeled into surgery. I am ready.

The phone rings and Mom answers, then hands it to me. I hear Dusa's reassuring voice, so confident. "You're going to be fine," she tells me, and I believe her.

The orderlies arrive to take me to the operating room, so Jeff leans over my gurney to give me a kiss. "This is it, hon," I say. "Yes, it is," he says, his voice subdued. His words say he is with me in my optimism, but his expression tells me he's cautious about overreaching, about expecting too much. Waving goodbye to my personal entourage—Jeff, Mom, my stepdad, and Liz—I'm wheeled from my room and down the hall.

I lie on the gurney, staring at the ceiling of the operating room. One by one the surgeons arrive. They offer me brief hellos and turn their attention to their colleagues. I stare up at them as they converse over my body, and I notice the underbellies of their chins, their hand gestures as they talk procedure. "Today's the day," I say, interrupting them. "What?" one says. They all look down at me. "Today's the day," I repeat. "Don't worry. Everything's going to be fine."

They seem amused by my confidence, my desire to reassure them, these titans of the knife. They shift from talking to me to talking about me, and I hear mention of the anesthesiologist having arrived.

"Are you ready, Lauren?" says a familiar voice. It's Bob. Even with his surgical cap and mask now in place, I recognize him. He has sincere eyes, the kind that tell me he really *does* want to know if I'm ready. No sooner do I nod my okay than I see the anesthesiologist moving toward my face with a hard plastic mask. I interrupt again.

"That crystal better be there when I wake up," I say, motioning to my right hand with my head because my arms are tied down. My tone says I'm kidding, but I'm not. The crystal had *better* be there when I come to. I hear a few courtesy chuckles as the mask covers my face and I slip away.

I hear Jeff's voice in the distance and blink my eyes several times to bring my vision into focus. I see my husband jogging toward me across a large room, skirting empty gurneys that create an obstacle course between the two of us, his expression one of genuine elation. Mom is behind him, and Bob behind her, both of them smiling. Because it's Saturday and there are no other surgical patients in the post-op area, the rules have been bent to allow my husband and mother a brief visit. I lie perfectly still on the gurney, thoughts beginning to take shape. It happened. I got my miracle.

"You did great, honey," Jeff says as he kneels next to me and takes my hand in his. I smile my response because forming words is too difficult. I'm still paralyzed by the anesthesia; my head feels heavy, my thinking fuzzy. Mom and Bob join Jeff and confirm that the surgery indeed went well. Jeff tells me to rest up and he kisses my forehead. I'm asleep again in no time.

"Mushrooms and green peppers."

"Pepperoni for me."

"I'll take pepperoni too." I recognize this last voice as belonging to my stepdad, and I'm now annoyed that my cocoon of comfort, the same feeling I have when awakening after a long stretch of sleep, has been dissolved.

"Shhhh," I say meekly and with Herculean effort, my eyes still closed. I hear subdued talk of moving to the hallway, familiar voices—Pam, Mom, Karen. I try to recapture that fuzzy warmth, the cottony sensation that embraced me between the waking world and sleep, just conscious enough to appreciate the supreme restfulness of this space. But all the talk of pizza orders has broken the spell. And because I'm familiar with the no-food-till-you-fart drill that follows surgery, I'm further annoyed that my postsurgical sleep was interrupted specifically by talk of food, food that I will not be permitted to enjoy.

I open my eyes and see that I'm back in my large corner room of the Transitional ICU. Mom tells me Dr. Brown pulled strings to hold this room for me while I was under the knife. It is these little demonstrations of kindness, the bending of hospital rules, the ignoring of nonessential protocol, that have helped my family and me feel the humanity that is all too often disguised in the high-tech environment of hospitals—specifically intensive care units, whose main function is swift intervention during acute crises rather than providing comfort.

Little handmade signs adorn the walls. One says *Good job, Wa! Nice healing!* Another, *My miracle came true!* And another, *My heart is filled with love and joy for you on this, your Miracle Day! Love, Sabra.* She always was the dramatic one among my core group of women friends, most of whom are as emotionally restrained as our collective corporate résumés would suggest.

Sabra's face comes into view as she leans in toward me. "Hey, girlie. How do you feel?"

"So rested," I whisper, not because I'm trying to keep the noise down but because it's the best I can do.

"I'm going to leave so you can sleep, but I'll be back again on Monday."

"I won't be here," I say, fully believing the words as they leave my mouth.

"Don't worry," she says. "I'll find you." I drift off again.

I awaken to see one of my regular nurses changing the dressing on my incision. As she pulls wads of gauze, now wet and bloody, from my lower abdomen, she begins describing the details of the surgery to me.

"Please don't," I say, hoping my voice conveys both patience and authority. "This is my miracle. You can talk medical details later." She nods her understanding and finishes repacking the opening in silence. I cling to my interpretation of the surgery's miraculous nature like a dog to a bone. My perspective defies logic, but logic alone won't explain why, in less than two weeks, I will go home.

"I'd like everyone to be quiet. Don't talk about the medical stuff in front of me," I tell Mom and Jeff after my nurse leaves. "Just focus on positive thoughts about my healing." Mom immediately makes a note to that effect and posts it on the door to my room for the hospital staff.

"This is *my* miracle," I say, squeezing my right hand around the crystal, still taped in place. Again, I sleep.

Hours later, I wake up and look around the room. Outside the window it's dark, the San Francisco night dotted with streetlights and illuminated buildings. My mother sits in the corner reading her book. We're alone.

"Mom? Could you tell me now what they did to me during the surgery?"

Tentatively, she shares one detail after another, pausing between each nugget of information to determine if I can handle more: the roughly four liters of loose blood that poured from my body when the incision was made; the removal of a six-liter blood clot in my lower abdomen; the additional pints of blood that were pumped into my body during the surgery; the four plastic tubes that now pierce my belly to facilitate further drainage of gunk.

My kidneys, the doctors feel, will improve as my liver function improves. My liver itself, however, remains an issue because, as Bob explained to Mom, it looked pretty beat up. I did not need a hysterectomy after all, she says, which disappoints me. Having a uterus means having the ability to get pregnant again. I never want to be pregnant again. I know this as clearly as I know my own name. I will not—*cannot*—go through this sort of nightmare again.

Mom describes how the surgeons held my uterus, my liver, my kidneys in their hands and, in effect, hosed off the toxic gunk that clung to them; how they vacuumed from my abdomen the fluids that didn't belong there; and finally, how the decision was made not to close the incision for fear of infection. Only the peritoneum—the sac that holds my guts—was stitched shut, leaving an eight-inch open surgical wound that

Mom refers to as "fillet of Lauren" and "the shark bite." This last piece of information bothers me. *My belly is still cut open?* I have a hard time imagining how this is possible, but when Mom offers to find a hand mirror so I can see for myself, I flatly refuse. Hearing about this shark bite is one thing. Seeing it, quite another.

Simply listening to all the details of the surgery has exhausted me, and now I want to sleep more. Before I drift off I silently will myself to dream about flying. I want to fly right out of this hospital, this situation, miracle or no miracle. I'm ready to fly. And fly I do, "pain-free and all over the place," I tell Mom after awakening later, a big smile on my face as I recount the details for her. Was it the lingering effect of the anesthesia? The power of suggestion? Or did my soul, the singular part of me that isn't broken, determine that it was time for a respite, however brief, from this shattered body I inhabit?

19

RAW. THAT'S HOW I FEEL WHEN I AWAKEN at four in the morning, sixteen hours after coming out of my third surgery in less than a month. Just plain raw.

I'm offered a shot of morphine and gladly accept. Once a proponent of riding out the worst headache rather than succumbing to the quick relief of medication, I'm now the pharmaceutical industry's biggest fan. Morphine, I've learned, offers more than a respite from physical pain. It also offers a respite from reality, including the reality of a long rehabilitation that I'd rather not think about yet.

My mother and sister run my body through a series of simple exercises. Under Karen's direction, they each cradle an arm, lift it in the air and return it to the air mattress. They repeat this cycle four times before they shift their focus to my legs, lifting each off the bed about a foot. As with my arms, five cycles are performed. Next, Karen instructs me to pump my feet as if stepping on the brakes of a car. I can't see my feet, but I suspect they are moving, if only a few inches. This is progress. We move to breathing exercises. Karen guides me through taking as full a breath as I can manage, which turns out to be a fraction of my lung capacity in the heyday of my life as an avid runner. I'm stunned by the difficulty of a simple deep breath, yet my sister praises my efforts. I find her words calming, reassuring. Absent is the acerbic humor and sarcasm that defined our sibling interactions for decades. For now, Karen is my teacher, nurse, and therapist, and her sole purpose in this moment is to nurture and encourage me. Wrapped in her cloak of comfort, I drift back to sleep in no time.

04/02/00—At 7:30 a.m., I had to chug down my morning supplements. I passed Karen a big bottle of water too. This was before Lauren could have any ice chips, and I acted without thinking. Karen and I almost choked on our water when we spotted Lauren, lying in bed, the third finger on each hand making obscene gestures at us. Funny. Unless you were the one who couldn't have any water.

At eight o'clock, a steady stream of specialists begins to flow in and out of my room. First is Keyser Söze, the obstetric surgeon with near-celebrity status among my regular team of doctors. I've been warned that he's "not much of a people person," that his elusive nature leads him to do most of his follow-up visits in the middle of the night when his surgical patients are likely to be sleeping. But here he is, inspecting the four grenade-like flasks that are connected to the drainage tubes protruding from my belly, which he inserted himself during my miracle surgery. He says little, but offers me a smile before he turns to leave.

Next is my obstetrician, who smiles and chats and shares encouraging test results. But I'm the one with few words now. My need to affix blame for not catching and preventing this preeclamptic nightmare remains strong, and she is my sole target. It will be years before I'll understand the insidious nature of preeclampsia and its ability to stay well below the surface of presenting symptoms until it is, all too often, too late. For now, I have no concept of how difficult early diagnosis can be, especially in cases like mine, which for the first eight months of my pregnancy showed none of the classic signs: no high blood pressure, no protein in the urine. For now, I remain attached to my need to dislike my OB, to hold her responsible. I feign fatigue to avoid a direct conversation and she soon departs.

The doctor in charge of the ICU visits next and declares that I seem to have turned a corner. I like his steady demeanor, surely a huge asset when it comes to handling the outsized egos that are certain to collide in the management of patients in an intensive care unit.

And my last visitor of the day is Dusa, every bit as much a healer as the medical experts with multiple degrees who visited earlier. She's here to do craniosacral work, and since this is my first experience with it, I have no idea what to expect. She cradles my head in her hands for five or ten minutes, then moves to the side of my body, where she slides one hand underneath me to support my sacrum. She alternates between these two locations for almost an hour, a few minutes at the sacrum, back to the head, and then back to the sacrum. The result is a sense of absolute peace.

When the craniosacral work is complete, Dusa pulls out her crystals and places them on specific areas of my body—meridian points, she calls them. She speaks of imagery techniques I can use during my physical therapy sessions. I tell her I feel like I no longer remember how to stand.

"Every cell in your body remembers how to stand, Lauren," she says. "Call on your brain cells to help you remember how to move." I believe her when she tells me I'll heal. As she prepares to leave, I extract a promise from her to return, and Mom follows her into the hallway to set up another appointment.

The following morning, Keyser Söze returns for another visit and once more inspects my drainage flasks, which the nurses empty whenever they reach capacity, about twice a day. The volume and color of the drained fluids looks good, he says. To me, it looks like thick cherry cola, but Keyser Söze seems pleased. So pleased, in fact, he comes back the next day. The nurses are impressed. He rarely visits a patient more than once during daylight hours, I'm told. In the meantime, Karen and I have made an interesting discovery. When I laugh, fluid drains more quickly from my body. The next time Keyser Söze appears in the doorway, Karen jumps from her seat and stands by my bed. "Hey, Doc, look what happens when I make her laugh," she says. Turning toward me, she tells stories of the ways we used to get in trouble together, does her decades-old imitation of the robot from *Lost in Space* episodes we watched as kids, and mentions several high school boyfriends, hers and mine, whose names alone are enough to elicit a comical response. I laugh, and as I do several of my drainage tubes noticeably spurt more gunk into their flasks. When I stop laughing, the output slows to a trickle.

"See? Laughter really is the best medicine," Karen says. Keyser Söze smiles, but it's clearly a courtesy smile. How many times before has this discovery been shared with him by the family members of his surgical patients? He continues his examination, applying pressure on my abdomen where the drainage tubes poke through my skin. His face remains expressionless.

"Is there anything I should be concerned about?" I ask.

He touches my hand while brushing a strand of hair off my face with his other hand. "Everything's okay," he says. "Everything will be fine." His modest demeanor and soft voice are reassuring. *Everything will be fine.* The mantra I repeated—no, demanded—while lying on the operating table during Clare's birth. Keyser Söze turns and leaves the room.

The next several days bring exponential progress in my physical recovery. Mom feels comfortable enough to go home again, to reconnect with her normal life in Boulder. With the help of morphine, I'm able to sit up and pivot from the bed to a chair, aided by several nurses. I spend two hours a day sitting in this chair, though the doctors would prefer six. I'm eating once more—a banana here, a bowl of miso soup there—despite a weak appetite. I manage to consume about 800 calories a day, though the doctors would prefer 2,400.

Bob stops by to tell me how well my organs are doing, much to his surprise. "And?" I say. He looks puzzled. So I point to my right hand. "My crystal! Let's give it some credit."

"I'm going to have all my patients do that," he says, laughing. And though I know he won't actually start taping crystals to the hands of his surgical patients, I appreciate his willingness to accept the integration of unconventional approaches into my treatment plan. Bob assures me that I'll be out of the Transitional ICU within a week. In fact, less than forty-eight hours later, I'm transferred to another step-down unit, the Critical Care floor.

My new room is palatial: a large corner suite with hardwood floors and expansive views of downtown San Francisco. As I'm wheeled in on my hospital bed, one of the nurses kids me about being a big shot because this room is reserved for VIPs. Or patients they really like. I assure her I'm not a VIP, nor has my hospital behavior earned me the title of Miss Congeniality. I learn that Bob's daughter was born in this room and that my obstetrician recovered from her hysterectomy in this room. And in this room, I will take my first walk in almost two weeks.

I'm given a shot of morphine to dull the pain that accompanies all movement. Jeff pulls me up to a sitting position and motions for a nurse to slide my legs off the side of the bed. He holds me, gently and on the few parts of my body that aren't bruised, until the vertigo passes. Without saying a word, Jeff is, I suspect, training my new team of nurses on the particulars of how best to physically maneuver my body. He's good at this, able to solidify the help and commitment of others without ever explicitly asking for or demanding it. It's a skill that works wonders in a hospital setting full of people who hurt, people like me.

My physical therapist, Amy, brings a walker to my bedside. A nurse gathers up the four drainage flasks and realizes the tubes attaching them to my belly aren't long enough for her to hold all four. She enlists the help of another nurse, and they each take two flasks in hand on either side of me. Amy and Jeff help me stand, Jeff's arms acting as a forklift under my armpits while Amy pushes from behind. I grip the sides of the walker and wait for my breathing to become steady. Someone puts another hospital gown on my body to cover my backside, then ties it around my neck like a cape. A third nurse joins our entourage and takes my IV pole in hand. Amy and Jeff release their grip on me but remain close, ready to grab me if I falter. Though dizzy, I am determined. *My doctors want me walking? I'll show them walking!*

I jerk the walker forward a few inches and slide my slippered feet across the smooth floor, my breathing labored. Congratulations are offered. *Way to go* from Amy. *Good job, honey* from Jeff. I do it again. Rest. Do it again. Rest. Two minutes later I'm at the doorway, and Jeff and Amy tense up. There's an inch-wide strip of rubber separating the hardwood flooring in my room from the thin institutional carpeting in the hallway. Amy squats, ready to assist my feet over the small bump if need be. I clear the hurdle without help, and our strange little parade continues its halting procession down the hallway. Despite my curiosity about these new surroundings, my gaze remains forward. Any eye movement left or right upsets my equilibrium, and I already feel as though I may vomit. I continue my determined shuffle toward my destination: the nurses' station twenty feet away.

Once there, I pivot, pausing to accept more congratulatory remarks from the nurses behind the desk before making my way back toward my room. Jeff's excitement is obvious. He jogs ahead of us, ducks into the room, and returns with the camera. "Smile," he says. I try to look up and face the camera, but dizziness forces me to shift my gaze downward, smiling nonetheless. I am walking. And I am—in this moment—happy, even optimistic about the future.

That evening, I lie in my hospital bed as Liz and Jeff review my latest numbers, which apparently aren't good. Their matter-of-fact demeanor annoys me. All this talk of numbers slipping, as if I've failed some ridiculous test I didn't even realize I was required to take. I don't want to be a part of this conversation, so I close my eyes and pretend to sleep. Jeff and Liz continue talking about me, and this pisses me off even more.

"Karen and Mom are more tuned in to my needs than you are," I tell Jeff after Liz leaves. He looks as if I've slapped him, but I continue, undaunted, through tears.

"I'm tired of having people talk about me! Especially right in front of me, eyes closed or not." Jeff is silent, his expression now blank.

"It's like there's a party going on around me and I'm not a part of it," I snap. Even I recognize that I'm trying to pick a fight with Jeff, but he refuses to engage. With just a few biting words from me, he has checked out.

04/05/00—This evening, Jeff said Lauren had beaten up on him. He said when it's time for Lauren to have dialysis, it's like talking with a six-year-old.

The following morning, Karen arrives to relieve Jeff for several hours. She offers me breakfast, but I refuse to eat, relying solely on my feeding tube. Bob stops by and tells me I need to eat real food in order to heal. I argue with him as well, telling him I'm getting plenty of nutrition from my feeding tube. He orders the tube removed.

When I'm transferred to the chair for my two hours out of bed, the process is more difficult than usual. It's as if none of my strength and determination of yesterday ever existed. Karen asks me if I'm okay and I slur my words in response. I'm lethargic and confused, and my legs are more swollen than usual—all signs that more frequent dialysis sessions are needed.

A few hours later, I lie covered in warm blankets as the portable dialysis machine slowly draws my entire blood supply through its filtering process, returning the cleansed blood back into my body. After the procedure, I'm able to enunciate my words, my voice is strong, and my conversations are refocused on recovery. I eat solid food again and later, when Karen insists that I use the toilet instead of the bedpan, I acquiesce. A nurse disconnects my IV line from the pole by my bed, and with the help of two people I'm pulled to standing. I shuffle to the bathroom using my walker, pivot, grip the safety bar on the wall, and lower myself onto a commode attachment that makes the toilet seat a foot taller than normal. Resting my arms and forehead on the walker, I sit for more than ten minutes, waiting for whatever will come out to do so. When I'm ready to return to bed, my strength is gone, so Karen pulls me up and wipes my bottom. I shuffle my way back to my bed, where a fresh pad has been placed on the middle of the mattress.

In preparation for her departure tomorrow, Karen establishes a routine for me, something she deems necessary for my current stage of recovery. She teaches Jeff how to pull me off the toilet and wipe my bottom. She coaches my new team of nurses on how best to interact with and motivate me. And she thoroughly exhausts me with this new regimen. I neither like nor appreciate her efforts. Yet I cry myself to sleep that night at the thought of losing her.

20

"TODAY'S THE BIG DAY," says my nurse. "You excited?"

"Yes," I say. "Can't wait."

I'm lying. The truth is, I'm not excited—I'm nervous. Tim and Dede are flying in from Orange County with Clare for a half-day visit and I don't know if the baby will like me. Will she snuggle with recognition in my arms? Or will she wail with confusion, crying *No! No! This is not my mother!* And I'm ashamed because I don't know if *I* will like the baby. If I hadn't gotten pregnant, I wouldn't be lying in this high-tech hospital bed, wouldn't have to listen to people tell me how lucky I am to simply be alive. What if I feel only resentment when I see her? Worse, what if I feel nothing? Because that's what I'm feeling right now. Nothing. And this makes me feel more shame than I've ever felt. I'm too exhausted to try to make sense of all these feelings and non-feelings, too exhausted even to think about Clare, the baby I wanted long before I became pregnant.

The nurse wants to change the dressing on my surgical wound, the first of three times today. A shot of morphine surges through my IV line as Jeff turns on the boom box to play the CD my cousin Chris made especially for me. It's a compilation of songs that are both unusual and calming, titled Lauren's Healing CD. I pick up my special crystal from the bedside table, hold it firmly in my right hand, and close my eyes, not wanting to see the mound of gauze, wet with blood, which the nurse removes from my lower abdomen. The music-morphine combination creates a tolerable environment, enabling me to focus my attention elsewhere, anywhere but here. Yet I still feel the tug of first-aid tape against bruises as it's pulled from the area surrounding my open surgical wound, the eerie sensation of movement within my belly as it's unpacked and repacked with gauze. Twenty minutes later the dressing change is complete, and I can now enjoy the dreamy state of numbness from the morphine without intrusion.

Around ten, a commotion in the hallway gets Jeff's attention. He rises to his feet looking perplexed, caught off guard. I recognize the familiar boom of my brother's voice as he and the hospital staff greet one another. Then, there it is: the sound of a baby mewing, followed by lots of cooing and *She's so beautiful* and *Look how big she is.* Now several nurses crowd my doorway giving me that look reserved for the guest of honor at a surprise birthday party. *Surprise! Now eloquently tell us all how happy you are about this emotional overload.* Tim enters my room, a broad smile on his face. Behind him is Pam, the self-appointed airport taxi. And behind Pam is Dede, holding my baby. My Clare.

"I thought you weren't coming until eleven!" Jeff snaps. Then he softens, his eyes watery from holding back tears. His exhaustion is showing, that hallmark demeanor of patience cracking. Rarely have I seen my husband short-tempered with others, diplomacy being one of his greatest assets. I have no idea how arduous this experience has been for him. My attention has been focused solely on me—*my* needs, *my* pain. Even now, with the frailty of his emotions so apparent, I'm unable to empathize.

Jeff composes himself and lifts our baby from my sister-in-law's arms, kissing the top of her head as he walks toward me. He hasn't held his daughter since the day he loaded her into Tim and Dede's rental car more than a month ago. Gently, reverently, he places Clare by my side, careful to keep her swaddled body away from my lower abdomen, while draping one of my arms around her. He doesn't let go until he's sure I have the strength to hold her without harming either of us. Everyone is watching, waiting. I stare at my baby girl's face. I sense they all want me to say something, to acknowledge the moment, but no words come. Only tears. And that is when I feel a certainty settle deep into my soul, as if Keyser Söze's comments yesterday were prophetic. *Everything will be fine.* And I know that it will be; that it already is.

I dote on Clare, play with her little fingers, and allow her to pump her pudgy legs against my hand. When she fusses, Dede pulls a bottle of warm soy formula from the diaper bag and positions it in my left hand at the angle my baby prefers. Her instructions are subtle, neither presumptive nor patronizing.

"Here you go, little one," I say, pretending it's the most natural thing in the world for me to be feeding my five-week-old baby for the first time. She takes the nipple and gulps down a full four-ounce bottle, and this alone gives me a bigger emotional boost than I've had since being pregnant. Maybe I'm not a complete failure as a mother after all. Maybe I *can* actually care for my daughter.

Just as I begin to feel the rhythm of motherhood, exhaustion envelops me. My eyelids flutter and my attention drifts toward the window, the door. Dede senses my need for a break and suggests that she take Clare for a walk. She leaves the room with my baby and—I'll later learn—leans against the corridor wall and breaks down, her relief at my survival overwhelming.

Lunch arrives, and I immediately reach for a notepad and pen from the bedside table. Tim and Jeff watch as I eat—a bite of sandwich here, a carrot stick there—slowly, cautiously, as if I'm forcing myself to do so, which I am. I pick up the pen and painstakingly write down what I've consumed before looking up its caloric value in the dietary reference book I insisted Jeff buy for me. I record the number of calories and any grams of protein in a column next to my list of food. I'm obsessed with proving to the doctors that I'm capable of eating 2,400 calories a day—their requirement for discharging me from the hospital. To date, I'm not even close to this goal, but I continue to obsess over each small bite.

"What's with the list?" Tim asks.

"I have to prove to the doctors that I've eaten enough," I say. My brother and husband exchange looks across my hospital bed. After eating less than 400 calories of food, I put my fork down, push the tray away, and cry.

"What's wrong, Wa?" Tim asks.

"I don't see much progress," I say. "I still feel so weak." Jeff and Tim stand on either side of my bed, each holding one of my hands.

"I can appreciate how you might feel that way," Tim says, his tone more compassionate now. "But in early March—and that's only a little more than a month ago—we all saw you near death. Now look at you! You can get in and out of bed, take short walks, eat regular food."

I continue crying.

"You've come so far from where you were. Don't beat up on yourself," Tim says.

I want to believe my brother, want to change my attitude, but when I lift my gaze to look him in the eye, I'm distracted by water—lots and lots of water—running down the far wall. And mist in the air. All around us, mist! Disbelief twists my facial expression. This can't be, can it?

"What is it?" Jeff asks. He's familiar with this look, knows it all too well.

I stall. There can't possibly be water running down the wall, but if I tell them what I see they won't let me go home. And I really want to go home. I keep quiet and look away from the watery wall.

"Do you see something, Wa?" There is an edge of tension—or is it fear?—in Tim's voice. He hasn't seen this yet: his sister, post-encephalopathy, slipping back into confusion. I'm crying harder now.

"Don't you see it?" I ask. "The water running down that wall? The mist in the air?" Jeff and Tim turn toward the far wall and back toward me. They both shake their heads.

"I'm sorry, Wa," Tim says. "There's nothing there."

Soon, I'm again hooked up to the dialysis machine, and afterward I no longer see the water or the mist.

04/08/00—Tim talked privately with Jeff and said, "You're the only person in this ordeal who isn't giving himself a break." Jeff said he really liked Karen's idea of having a nurse's aide take over the daytime duties. When Tim asked, "What are you going to do for Jeff? Define what you're going to do for yourself or you won't be good for anybody." Jeff replied, "Right now, I don't think I'm good for anybody anyway."

Keyser Söze stops by and snips the four plastic flasks from their drainage tubes, leaving about six inches of each tube hanging from my belly. He takes notice of Clare, now napping on the bedside cot, and compliments her beauty before leaving.

I have to use the bathroom, so I struggle to pull myself up using the triangular bar overhead. Dede grips my arms to steady me while I sit on the edge of the bed catching my breath and waiting for the vertigo to pass.

"Mom said I was a Capricorn, a goat, and that I'm climbing up a mountain," I say, not realizing that she told me this while I was comatose. "But I don't know how high the mountain is and I feel like I'm in a fog." In Dede's presence the tears come easily and without embarrassment. She's been with me through a number of upsetting ordeals, from breaking off a three-year relationship to Spike getting hit by a car while I was traveling on business. She knows me well, understands when to nurture and when to nudge.

"You know, Lauren, I was here five days after Clare was born," Dede says. "You were hooked up to so many machines, and we were talking with the liver transplant team. You saw me and you even held Clare, but you probably don't remember it."

"You're right. I don't."

"So in my opinion," she says, "you're now three-quarters of the way up that mountain. Only one-quarter to go."

Encouraged by her assessment, I reach for my walker and *climb*—from bed. As I stand, the drainage tubes that no longer attach to flasks dangle from my belly and fluid pours from them. Dede and I both look from the small puddles on the floor to each other and laugh.

Later that afternoon the time comes for Tim, Dede, and Clare to leave for the airport, so my brother collects the baby gear scattered about the room. Dede lifts Clare from my bed, where she's tucked into my right arm, sound asleep. I avert my gaze so I won't have to see my little girl being taken away, again.

"Goodbye," I say. Dede walks back toward me, Clare's head nestled against a burp cloth on her shoulder.

"Can we just say *See you later?*"

21

AT MY REQUEST, PATRICIA ARRIVES AT NOON. Jeff rises from his chair, crossing the room to shake her hand. Elegantly dressed in a pantsuit, her shoulder-length hair neatly styled, she appears much younger than her fifty-some years. Jeff hasn't seen Patricia since she counseled him through his fears of fatherhood seven months ago. He looks relieved, with that subtle brightening of his expression I've noticed whenever someone arrives, allowing him another brief furlough—a walk around the block, a coffee break in the lobby.

Today, Patricia is here for me. It's been a year and a half since she helped me with issues that arose from making a career change motivated solely by money. Most nights, I drove home from work past ten o'clock, crying with frustration. I'd pull into the garage of our rental home, where Jeff often met me with a hug and a glass of red wine. But once a week, I'd leave work earlier than usual, six o'clock, and drive to Patricia's office to spend an hour in her calming presence. Combining her MD in psychiatry with her highly developed intuition, she'd help me connect with the expansiveness of my life beyond the confines of the workplace, and with each visit I felt restored.

Approaching my bed, Patricia seems astonished by my appearance. Gone is the slim, attractive businesswoman whose strength once shone through despite her sorrows. In her place is an oversized, jaundiced sick person she barely recognizes. Sitting in the chair Jeff has brought over for her, she lightly squeezes my forearm in greeting and then hands me a small gift. I fumble with ribbons and tissue paper until I uncover a delicate stained-glass angel ornament. Her wings are spread wide, her hands cupped together and held upward as if handing something to a higher source. *Here,* she seems to be saying, *please fix this.* I thank Patricia and hand the angel to my husband for safekeeping.

After Jeff leaves, Patricia tries to engage me in a conversation about my feelings regarding the illness, my baby, my relationship with Jeff. But I don't want to talk about my feelings. As far as I'm concerned they're not important. I have my own agenda with Patricia, the real reason for requesting a visit. I want answers. And I want her to provide them not with the abilities that earned her a fancy degree, but with her less publicized psychic skills.

"How long will it take me to recover?" I ask point blank. She hesitates, as if weighing how much truth I can handle.

"It could take a year," she replies.

"Okay," I say. I'm not sure what I think of this prediction. A year sounds like a long time. Intellectually, I know that I'll make noticeable progress in no time at all; already have. But a year? That's a long time. I move on to my next question.

"Why does it feel like my soul isn't inside my body?" I ask.

I make no attempt to explain what I mean by this question. It is as simple as it sounds: My body feels vacant, my soul off somewhere else. Patricia gazes past me, as if there is someone standing behind me with whom she is conferring. I remember this look from several of my sessions with her in the past. When she held my gaze, I knew I was dealing with Patricia the MD. When she looked slightly past me, she was Patricia the intuitive. Clearly, I'm interacting with the latter.

"Because it isn't," she responds. "Your soul is around you, but not completely in you. Most of it is hovering off to the side of your body."

"How do I get it back inside my body?" I ask. Patricia laughs. "Lauren, there's a good reason it's outside of your body. For now, it must be." She senses my confusion and continues her explanation. "Your soul is such a powerhouse, so high energy, that if it settled completely back into your body right now, it would short-circuit your physical being, much like an overcharged electrical circuit. Your body is broken and must strengthen itself before it can handle all the strength of your soul. And your soul understands that, so it's standing off to the side until your body is ready. Does that make sense?"

It does. It completely resonates with the feelings I've been having lately, feelings that I'm not fully here.

04/10/00—Lauren can tell her brain isn't right yet. She's very weak. Face, arms, and legs are thin to gaunt. Still has a huge belly that she says "looks like Sally Struthers should be talking about me on a public service announcement."

With the help of antidepressants, I have another restful night of sleep. Jeff, however, does not. He sleeps on the cot in my room and awakens with a stiff back. But he knows that help is about to arrive, and at nine o'clock the private nurse hired by Tim knocks at my door, then lets herself in. Ola is tall—almost six feet—and looks strong despite her age, which I estimate to be early sixties. She wears scrubs with a bright print, and her hair is pulled back in a bun. She smiles and shakes hands with Jeff before addressing me. Her manner is both professional and warm. I don't like her.

Oh, I'm sure she's a nice person and has friends and family who love her. But she's been hired as a replacement for Jeff, his relief pitcher. And I don't want a relief pitcher. I want Jeff. And even as I think those words, I realize that I'm lying to myself.

This isn't about me wanting Jeff by my side, because very often when he is I respond with petulance to anything he says. No, this is about Jeff *not* wanting to be by my side. He wants to leave me with this stranger, this hired friend and helper.

I can't blame him for wanting a break from me. He has borne the brunt of my anguish over this illness, all these feelings that whip me around, sending me in different emotional directions at the slightest shift in current. Grateful one minute, incensed the next. Amused and laughing one minute, depressed and crying the next. Like a sponge, Jeff has absorbed these emotional jags despite warnings from nurses and family members to put more effort into his own self-preservation. For as long as I have known him, Jeff has always been the guy who sacrifices himself for those he loves. He is the guy for whom the "put your mask on first" airline messages were created because he's the guy who would never think to put his mask on before helping me with mine. It's a quality of Jeff's that I find both endearing and infuriating. He would sacrifice himself for me if I asked him to. But I don't.

Instead, I slowly erode his steadfast exterior, picking away at his loyalty one snipe at a time. "That's not the book I asked for!" I barked after he returned from another trip home at my request. I heard the bitchiness in my words even as they left my mouth, felt the unfairness of it all. I saw the change in my husband's disposition, the sadness on his face as the weeks passed and I continued to erratically dump on him. He now has a look of resignation, a look that says *I will prove my love for you by losing myself.*

But still.

I cannot bring myself to simply tell Jeff that I love him, that I appreciate all he has done for me, that I know how important it is for both of us to recover from this shared nightmare we've survived but not yet put behind us. And I don't know why I continue to hurl all my anger at him, why I behave so childishly about something that's not his fault. I turn my cheek for his kiss goodbye and avoid eye contact as he leaves.

Ola offers to give me a sponge bath or fluff my pillows or do whatever might make me more comfortable. I respond with brief noncommittal answers. Not exactly curt, but not engaging. She follows my cues and sits quietly in the corner with her book as I pretend to nap.

The following morning Jeff's mother, Bev, and his sister, Val, arrive from Michigan. Bev walks into my hospital room with a slight waddle and a bit of obvious discomfort. The two steel rods that were permanently placed in her back when she broke it three years ago have changed her gait. Val enters behind her, taking small cautious steps and using the wall to steady herself. When I saw Val over the Christmas holidays, her balance was much better. But when she's overly stressed she loses another increment of mobility. Clearly, her MS has gained ground as a result of my illness.

"Sorry, Wa, but you're down to visits from the C Team," Val jokes, referencing their respective medical challenges.

Jeff is with them, carrying my laptop under his arm. While I introduce Val and Bev to Ola, Jeff sets the computer on my bedside table and connects it to the hospital telephone line. First stop—E-trade. I've heard some discussion of the Silicon Valley crash that happened while I was comatose, and I want to check the balance of my 401(k). While pregnant, I invested in high-risk tech stocks with a lot of bravado and not much restraint. Like my body, they're now ravaged and we've lost tens of thousands of dollars in less than a month. I should be feeling upset or panicked or at least a bit nervous, but I'm surprisingly neutral about this discovery.

"*C'est la vie,*" I say to Jeff. He too is remarkably nonplussed by the loss of value in our accounts.

"Hey, we've been through worse," he says. Despite the smile on his face, the weariness in his eyes underscores the truth of this statement.

"Your insurance company has been making noise," my kidney doctor says when he stops by that afternoon to check on me. "They want to know why we're still keeping you at the hospital when all your surgeons have released you."

"What do you mean?" I ask, feeling my heartbeat quicken. My disdain for hospital life is overshadowed only by my sense of vulnerability in *not* having all the hospital staff around. How will Jeff care for me at home? What if medical help is needed? What if Spike jumps on me? I can feel the panic mounting, but I keep it from this doctor, as I still dislike him for his dearth of bedside manner. I will my facial expression to remain neutral.

"They're pushing us to send you to a rehab facility because it's cheaper than keeping you here." I remain silent. "You *don't* want to go to a rehab facility," he adds.

No, I don't. I've already been to a rehab facility, plenty of them. For the past three years, Spike and I have been volunteering with the local SPCA's pet-therapy program. Each week, I would load Spike into the car and drive to our assigned location—hospitals, nursing homes, and rehab facilities—to allow for patient interaction with a friendly furry animal. We'd spend two hours knocking on doors, visiting people in their rooms or in the community area, Spike entertaining them with tricks or resting her head on their laps and soaking in all the caresses and attention. The physical conditions of these institutions, especially those in poor neighborhoods, were often as dismal as the circumstances that brought their occupants to them: dimly lit hallways, sparse furnishings, an overabundance of plastic plants and flowers all coated with dust, and alarmingly low nurse-to-patient ratios. All too often I found a resident sitting alone in a dark room, or smelled the stench of an uncollected food tray hours after lunchtime, or saw signs of personal hygiene neglected: dirt under overgrown fingernails, the crust of dried saliva in the corner of a mouth.

I loathe the idea of being sent to a rehab facility.

"What are our options?" Jeff asks. His wrinkled brow tells me similar thoughts have run through his mind. Last Thanksgiving Jeff accompanied Spike and me on an all-day assignment, spending time at several different rehab facilities in the poorest neighborhoods of San Francisco, where most of the people we visited had no family members with whom to share the holiday. Afterward, we ate burgers and fries at a nearly empty diner in the Castro district and spoke of how grateful we were to have the financial means and family relationships that would prevent us from ever being in the situations of the people we had met that day.

"I doubt your insurance company will cover in-home care," my doctor says, speaking directly to Jeff. "But assuming you have the money to pay for nurses, I would highly recommend that we send her home. Most patients recover more quickly in their own environment."

Again I feel the acceleration of my heartbeat, the internal struggle of conflicting emotions. I want to go home. I don't want to go home. I hate the hospital. I need the hospital. But I definitely, beyond a doubt, do not want to go to a rehab facility.

"Home it is," says Jeff. "We'll find a way to make it work." His tone is neither reassuring nor dour.

"Okay, then," the doctor says. "I'll make sure her discharge orders include the equipment you'll need: wheelchair, handicap commode, stuff like that. You can pretty much set up what a rehab facility would offer right in your home. We'll give you a prescription for in-home physical therapy and home-care nurses, and then you'll just have to see how much insurance is willing to cover."

"Can I have a bed too? Like this one?" I ask. I feel as if I'll cry if he tells me no, can already feel the tears welling up. My belly, sides, arms, and bottom are covered in bruises, and the lightest pressure on any part of them creates a throbbing sensation as if I've been punched. Even my bones feel bruised from within. Everything hurts, inside and out. I want this air mattress that cushions every shift in position. I want this triangular monkey bar overhead that gives me something to grip when I move. I want these buttons that gently elevate my back or legs to increase my comfort. I want—no, *need*—this bed.

"I'll write a prescription for the bed too," my doctor says, and for the first time, I find myself softening toward him. Not much. He still has the outward warmth of a polar ice cap. But his willingness to let me have my bed suggests more tenderness than his manner implies. Somewhere under that armor of restraint from years as a surgeon is a guy who still cares.

22

THIS IS IT: THE DAY I'VE ANTICIPATED, fantasized about, begged for, even threatened a few doctors to get to. I'm leaving. Not to a step-down unit. Not to a quieter room down the hall. This is the real deal. Home.

A nurse I don't recognize explains my discharge orders to Jeff: each medication's dosage, how often the home-care nurse will visit to change the dressing on my still-open wound, how often he must give me the Epogen shots to rebuild my red blood cell count.

Shots? What shots?

"Don't worry," she says, noticing my anxiety. "After all you've been through, this is nothing."

Nothing? What does she know? Another needle—this *nothing*—scares the hell out of me. I bite my lip to keep my emotions in check, but when someone calls the nurse into the hallway I fall apart, on this, my discharge day. My illness has transformed me from a strong-willed optimist to a frightened deer, jittery at every small shift in my surroundings or plans. This is but one more example of the new me. Jeff holds my hand and reassures me in a tone that doesn't sound very reassuring. He too has changed.

The discharge nurse returns and tells Jeff that since he'll be giving me my shots he should practice on an orange to get the feel of injecting a needle. There's no way he's giving me shots.

"Betsy will show you how to do it," she says, as another nurse I don't recognize enters the room. Middle-aged and looking frazzled, Betsy forgoes any pleasantries and quickly demonstrates how to fill a needle, holding it up to the light and flicking it with her thumb and middle finger once it's full. With no understanding of how sensitive my body has become, she grips my upper right arm, causing me to cry harder than I already am. Thin and bruised, my arms have no muscle tone and very little flesh. Disregarding my tears, she plunges the needle into my upper arm, her message abundantly clear. *Buck up, lady.*

Later that morning, Bev arrives to help with the move home. She takes down photos, mostly of Clare, the baby I've spent less than five hours with since her birth six weeks ago. I suspect they were hung as a reminder that I'm now a mother and have a responsibility to pull through. Death is no longer an option. Bev quietly moves about the room collecting other items that were brought in to make hospital life more bearable: my boom box, several CDs of meditative music, cards and letters from well-wishers. She stacks everything on a cart someone delivered earlier and then unwinds the string of tiny white Christmas tree lights and the celestial garland that Pam wrapped around the bar over my bed. These too will go home with me.

A critical care intern enters the room. "I heard you're leaving us. Guess we'd better remove that dialysis port," he says. Fumbling with the ties of my hospital gown, he lowers it just enough to expose the small square box that was semipermanently installed in my chest near my clavicle. I find his small display of decency humorous because I doubt I'll ever be modest again. All of my immediate family and Jeff's immediate family—not to mention dozens of nurses and doctors—have seen every inch of my naked body. What's a little breast exposure during my final hours of incarceration?

He snips the stitches that hold the port in place and asks me to take a deep breath. I try to oblige but can only manage a shallow gasp, my lung capacity still severely limited. Exhaling, I feel a weird sensation in my chest, not quite pain, but mild discomfort. I've learned to keep my eyes closed tight during procedures, believing it best not to fully understand what's happening until afterward.

When he's finished, I open my eyes. The intern is smiling, my dialysis port and its long thin wire dangling from one of his gloved hands.

"You won't need that anymore either," he says, nodding toward the intravenous PICC line in my left arm, which was installed when it became clear that I'd be staying for a while. Snip, snip, snip. I feel another strange sensation as it's removed from my arm, and again I open my eyes to inspect the results. I scratch the area where the PICC line was, smearing tiny beads of blood across my forearm.

There's a knock at the door, and I look up to see an orderly in blue scrubs pushing a wheelchair into the room. As if on cue, Jeff and I both laugh. Covered with blankets, I look fairly small, even birdlike, as my feet, arms, neck, and face have lost most of their meatiness. There's no collagen left in my upper lip, so when I smile, I look like a freakish Halloween ghoul with bulging eyes and a creepy stretched-out mouth, a look Jeff has nicknamed Skeletor. But under the blankets I'm large, with a midsection twice the size it used to be.

"There's no way this ass is going to fit in that chair," I say. The orderly leaves to find something bigger.

There's another knock at the door and in walks Bob, wearing regular street clothing, his white medical coat noticeably absent. He's officially on vacation, he tells us, but didn't want to miss a personal farewell on the big day. He pulls up a chair and stays for half an hour, talking about everyday things, normal nonmedical things. When Bob gets up to leave, Jeff shakes his hand and promises to set a follow-up appointment for two weeks from now.

The orderly returns looking sheepish, almost apologetic, as he pushes an extra-wide wheelchair into the room. It looks like a small love seat. Instead of being insulted, I'm grateful because the bruised flesh that runs up and down my sides won't have to be squeezed against the arms of the chair. I thank him profusely and he tips an imaginary hat as he turns to leave.

Jeff helps me sit up, then holds onto me while we wait for the vertigo to pass. He removes my hospital gown as if undressing a newborn and slips a maternity nightgown over my head—the goofy but comfortable cow-print one I bought months ago as a joke, a reflection of how I felt as my body transformed itself into my baby's personal milk factory. But this milk factory never kicked into full production. My body became toxic. My baby left town. And my breasts seemed to understand that the plan had changed. They quickly dried up and shrank.

Jeff slides slippers onto my feet and helps me stand. Walker firmly in hand, I inch my way toward the wheelchair. Jeff puts a bed pillow on the black vinyl seat of the chair and then turns toward me. I need help getting situated and he's the only person I trust with this task because he understands how crucial a gentle grip is. He moves behind me and puts his arms under my armpits, carefully lowering me onto the pillow. My nurse tucks a large absorbent pad under my thighs and bottom, as my body still spurts little bits of waste wherever I sit. She adjusts my nightgown while Jeff lifts my deadweight legs onto the footrest.

A husky man carrying a clipboard ducks his head through the doorway. The embroidered name badge on his white shirt reads *Ed*.

"Larsen?" he asks, looking at his clipboard.

"That's me," I say.

"I'm from Mike's Mobile Medical Transport. Are you ready to go home?"

"Ready?" Jeff asks me.

I feel the same way I did after crossing the finish line of every marathon I've ever run—exhausted, but overwhelmingly pleased with myself for simply having survived.

"That's it?" I ask one of the nurses. My voice is weak, my breathing labored from the effort of getting settled in the wheelchair. "I can go home now?"

"Yep," she says. "You can go home."

Jeff walks alongside my wheelchair as Ed slowly pushes it toward the bank of elevators, my mother-in-law following closely behind with the cart. People in scrubs and white coats give us a wide berth as we pass. I feel like the homecoming queen in a small-town parade, my eyes brimming with tears of giddy anticipation. The desire to thank everyone who helped me get to this day envelops me, but since I don't remember most of them I simply flash my best Skeletor smile at everyone we see.

"I don't know if you treated me," I say, "but if you did, thank you. I'm going home."

Most smile down at me as if I'm a small child. In a sense I am. This is my do-over. I'm starting my life again.

As I'm wheeled off the elevator on the ground floor of the hospital, it all feels a bit anticlimactic. I expected more fanfare, perhaps a gathering of hospital staff waiting at the elevators, smiling, clapping in acknowledgment of our shared triumph. But they're off saving other lives, speaking in hushed tones to other people's families.

We reach the hospital lobby and I'm at once struck by the phenomenon of everyday life—people in regular street clothes, coming and going, talking, laughing. I'm amused by the stares I receive from all these normal-looking people, what with my deep yellow skin, drawn face, extra-wide wheelchair, and silly cow-print nightgown. We get within range of the automatic door sensor and *whoosh!* The sliding doors of the main hospital entrance part. Ed pushes my wheelchair into a beautiful clear April day. Closing my eyes, I tilt my head upward to feel the sun directly on my face. The everyday noises of city life surround me: the clanging of a distant cable car, someone whistling for a cab, the honking of car horns. I breathe in the first fresh air I have felt in my lungs for six weeks and one day, and its impact is overwhelming.

Glorious, I think. Absolutely *glorious.*

Part Two

Help me, Clarence, please. Please, I want to live again.

—GEORGE BAILEY, *It's a Wonderful Life*

23

MY EXTRA-WIDE WHEELCHAIR and I are strapped into a white van with a large Mike's Mobile logo on the exterior. Ed is in the driver's seat to my left, and his coworker, Tyson, is on the bench seat behind us, watching the floor mounts that hold my wheelchair in place to make sure they remain secure. Jeff and Bev follow us in the SUV.

I already trust Ed implicitly. He didn't smirk or roll his eyes when I explained how sensitive my body is, or when I implored him to drive slowly and carefully to avoid any jarring. Instead, he suggested we take Divisadero instead of Fillmore, even though it's a slightly longer route through the city to my home in Noe Valley.

"Bigger road, fewer potholes," he said.

Despite the joy of going home, the act of simply getting there has me more nervous than I'm willing to admit. I've gotten used to my hospital confinement, the bed, the lack of movement. Now I have hills to brave, turns to survive, stops and starts at intersections to endure. I hold my breath as we reach the second stoplight and slowly turn left onto Divisadero Street. Nothing. No pain. My body relaxes, not completely, but enough. I'm going to be okay.

Turning my attention toward the sights of the city, *my* city, I'm surprised by how much emotion wells up within me as we drive past landmarks I've seen on numerous drives through San Francisco in the past. "This is amazing," I say over and over again, as if I were a tourist visiting for the first time. Ed smiles every time I repeat myself. He's probably transported many patients from the hospital to their homes and seen this response often. I haven't allowed myself many thoughts of life before illness, didn't want my homesickness to intensify my overall sadness, so I kept my focus on life in the hospital. But today is different. I bask in the feeling of reclaiming my life, my city, my home.

We pass the odd little Church of Coltrane, a dilapidated storefront that's tucked between two commercial enterprises and dedicated to the music of one of my husband's favorite jazz musicians. Jeff and I have passed this church a hundred times, always telling one another we ought to check it out someday. Now I wonder why, in all the years we've lived here, we've never gone there.

On the left is Phuket Thai Restaurant. "Fuck it," I say.

"What?" Ed replies.

I point to the restaurant as the van idles at the stoplight. "Fuck it," I say again. "That's what we call it." Ed laughs.

As Divisadero turns into Castro, more signs of home come into view. On the right is Marcello's, where Jeff and I walked for pizza whenever we were too tired to cook, Spike always waiting patiently outside the restaurant for our leftovers.

"Best pizza in town," I say. As we drive past, a hospital memory surfaces: a hallucination in which Liz and I were in an office building (my ICU room) waiting for the elevator (the wall in front of my bed). Jeff and his dad were waiting outside in a cab (they weren't) so we could all go to Marcello's for pizza. I remember being impatient because the longer it took for the elevator to come, the greater the cab fare would be. How many more of these surreal flashbacks, I wonder, will emerge when I least expect them?

We drive up the steep hill that divides the Castro district from Noe Valley. Ed turns left on 21st Street, crosses Noe Street, and hangs a left onto Rayburn. I'm one block from home and the anticipation is almost too much. I think of Dorothy waiting to board the wizard's hot-air balloon. Might something go wrong to divert my trek home?

Ed turns the corner onto Liberty. "Right here," I say. "This is it."

I motion him into the first driveway. Jeff pulls past us and parks in an open spot on the street. Tyson opens the large sliding door on the side of the van, unhooks the floor mounts from my wheelchair, and begins to wheel me backward toward the ramp that Ed has activated from the driver's seat.

"Wait! Hold on a minute, please," says Jeff, as he jogs up to the van. "Would you mind waiting for a minute while I run inside and get the video camera?"

"Sure thing," Tyson replies, sitting back on his heels.

"Sorry," I say.

"No problem," Ed says, chuckling.

Jeff returns, holding the camcorder I gave him when we got engaged. "Okay, go ahead and bring her out of the van," he says, as if he's a film director and we're his cast. "Great, great," he says, slowly stepping backward, the camera covering half his face. "Smile, honey."

I shake my head as if embarrassed, when in truth I'm grateful, thrilled that he hasn't completely fallen apart from this ordeal. Amazed, really. I wave to the camera as I come down the ramp and shield my eyes from the bright sunlight as Tyson wheels me to the fifteen steps leading to our front door. Ed and Tyson look at the stairs, look at my 205-pound body, look at each other. We all laugh.

"Sorry," I say again.

"No problem," Ed replies, flexing his biceps in mock bravado.

Bev scoots past my wheelchair with another armload of my belongings, and Val watches from the top of the stairs, gripping the railing with both hands.

"On three," Ed says to Tyson, and on the count of three, I'm hoisted into the air, wheelchair and all. Sweat beads on their foreheads as they struggle toward the entrance, pausing between each step to catch their breath. I notice that the flowerboxes lining the stairway are filled with bright flowers—red and purple and yellow pansies surrounding French lavender plants, the same kind Jeff and I surrounded ourselves with when we were married in a rustic outdoor amphitheater. These same flowerboxes were filled with dead and decaying plants when I left for the doctor's office six weeks ago, but Jeff has thought of every detail, every small way he can say *Welcome Home*. The irony of the flowerboxes now brimming with new life is not lost on me.

With sweat streaming down their faces, Ed and Tyson set me down inside the front door. Bev pushes me farther into the living room and I immediately notice that the house is spotless. A vase of purple irises sits on the dining table. The French doors leading to our patio are open, revealing more flowerboxes overflowing with lavender and pansies. Spike stands at a slight distance from me, freshly groomed, tentatively wagging her tail. A homely maroon lift chair, the kind whose advertisements show old people being elevated to standing, sits in the corner where Jeff's reading chair used to be. "Day by Day," the song my friend Carrie and I jokingly sang to one another a year ago while dealing with an untenable work situation, is playing on the stereo, another of Jeff's carefully crafted homecoming details. I scan the room, the expectant faces of Val, Bev, and Jeff, from behind the camera, watching me. It's all too much. I drop my head in my hands and weep at the joy of returning home, the sadness of what was lost.

Jeff sets the camera down and kneels beside my wheelchair, folding me into his arms. He too is crying. Spike moves closer and nudges my arm with her snout. I look up to see Bev with her arm around Val, their cheeks wet with tears. I glance at the front door, where Ed and Tyson stand waiting for a signature on some paperwork, and notice that Ed is wiping his eyes with the back of his hand. Leaning into Jeff's neck, I allow a sense of absolute relief to wash over me.

I am home.

04/14/00—Lauren told Jeff to take down her list of goals for the year 2000. She told him she was simply going to "go with the flow." She told him that everything that's happening is supposed to be happening. Don't question it. We're right where we're supposed to be in our lives.

Trying my new lift chair for the first time, I sit atop two pillows to further soften its padded seat. Jeff tucks more fluffy goose-down pillows around me like Styrofoam peanuts encasing a delicate piece of china. Bev drapes a blanket over my lap, then wraps it snugly around my legs, while Jeff arranges an afghan around my shoulders like a shawl. I experiment with the buttons on the armrest, moving the chair forward and back, leg-rest up and down, until I find the most comfortable settings. Once the chair is adjusted, Spike moves in closer. Jeff holds her collar as a precaution, ensuring she won't suddenly leap onto my lap. I know she won't. On numerous occasions, I've watched my barely trained dog morph from irreverent to angelic simply by walking into the hospital room of an elderly patient, have seen that she somehow understands the need to be gentle, as if declaring *Hey, I may be a trash-can-tipping, kitchen-countertop-raiding troublemaker, but I'm not stupid!* Spike sets her head in my lap and I massage the top of her velvety body. She feels like home.

Val settles onto the couch across from me and Jeff helps her get comfortable as well—a pillow under her legs, a blanket around her shoulders. As daylight wanes, so too does Val's energy. This is my husband at his best. I watch him tend to his big sister and recall the weeks of sadness, the despair he felt after

Val's MS diagnosis four years ago. I remember how he sat in his reading chair in the darkened living room staring at nothing, and when I found him there I wrapped my arms around his broad shoulders. No words came to mind, so I said nothing as he whispered *I don't know what to do* over and over again. It was the first time I'd ever seen my then-fiancé cry.

Although Val rested at home earlier this afternoon while Bev and Jeff were at the hospital for my discharge, I can see that she's drained. My mother-in-law hands us each a mug of herbal tea and returns to the kitchen to prepare dinner.

"Thanks, Wa," Val says.

"What for?" I ask.

"I'm so tired of being the center of the family medical drama. I appreciate you taking the spotlight for a while."

"Happy to help."

We lift our mugs in a facetious toast.

A half hour passes and the smell of fish in the skillet overwhelms my senses. Food and I are still trying to reestablish our relationship, and my mouth, tongue, and throat remain coated with thrush. The combination of these factors makes me feel woozy and nauseated.

"I think I need to lie down," I say. "I'm a little tired." I'm lying, but I don't want to insult Bev, whose presence has given my husband a much-needed boost. Clearly, I'm not the only one in need of nurturing.

Jeff positions my walker in front of me as I fumble with the lift chair controls, raising the chair to its highest position. I steady my hands on the armrests and will myself to stand, but nothing happens. I try again. Nothing. There is a moment of silence as Val, Jeff, and Bev all wait to gauge my response.

"I got nothing," I say, laughing. Jeff moves to the back of the chair and slides his hands under my butt.

"On three," he says. "One, two, three!" And up I go the final six inches to standing. Val claps. Jeff lets out a sigh. And Bev offers a *bravo!* from the kitchen. Using my walker, I make my way down the short hallway, pausing at the entrance to the small second bedroom. Someone has moved the guest bed to the opposite side of the room, where my desk was the last time I was in this room. Tim and Dede's old crib, which Jeff and I brought home during our last drive to Orange County, stands fully assembled where the bed was. Brown cardboard shipping boxes and gift boxes covered in pastel baby-themed wrapping paper are stacked on the floor, the bed, even inside the crib.

"What's all that?" I ask Jeff.

"People sent gifts," he says. "I didn't want to open them without you."

"Wow," I say, feeling overwhelmed as much by others' kindness as by the thought of all the thank-you notes that will need to be written. I continue toward the master bedroom, where Jeff helps position me properly in my hospital bed, pulling a sheet looser here, fluffing up a pillow there.

"All set?" he asks.

"All set."

He kisses my forehead and returns to the living room. I look around our bedroom. The bookshelf, meditation table, and Spike's old worn ottoman, which she sits on to watch the action outside the window, are all gone, making room for my hospital bed and a hospital table on wheels. Jeff has hung the framed marathon photo on the wall by my bed. Next to it are a few photos of Clare, held to the wall with Scotch tape. The little white lights and shimmery garland from Pam have been restrung around the bars of my new bed. The door to the tiny half-bathroom is open, and I can see the medical commode dominating the little space. Everything else is as it was six weeks ago: the chunky wooden queen-size bed with its forest-green velvet duvet, the plain cream-colored curtains hanging from rustic metal rods with curlicues at each end, the earth-toned Berber carpeting that we installed when we rented this place because I didn't like the idea of walking barefoot on someone else's old carpeting. It's a simple look that permeates the house, yet now it seems richer, more comforting, like a sacred space I'm rediscovering. Spike's squeaky toys, usually littered all over the bedroom floor, are neatly piled in a corner. The sliding doors to the closet are partway open, and I see that it's still crammed with my old collection of business suits and my newer collection of maternity clothing, neither of which will ever be worn by me again.

Ten minutes pass, and Bev comes into my room carrying an oversized dinner plate piled high with rice, spinach, and codfish. "Did you want to eat in here?" she asks. Her voice is soft and comforting. I nod my head and discreetly hold my breath as she sets the plate on the rolling table.

"What would you like to drink?"

"Water's fine," I say, trying not to appear repulsed. Just looking at this enormous plate of food is overwhelming. The thought of even one bite of fish or spinach is revolting, but my desire to be polite overrides my desire to be honest. Lately I've been sensing the burden this illness has put on my family and friends, and I know how hard it must've been for Bev to come to California. Other than for our wedding, she's done no airline travel since breaking her back. She leaves the room to get my drink, but it's Jeff who returns, glass of water in hand. I immediately begin crying.

"What's wrong, honey?" he asks.

"I can't eat this. I don't want to be rude, but I can't eat this." I'm almost hyperventilating with anxiety.

"It's okay, it's okay," he says. "Mom'll understand."

"No!" I say. "Don't tell her. Just flush some of it down the toilet and take the plate back. *Please.*" Jeff is clearly perplexed by my fear of insulting Bev, but I insist and he complies. Five minutes later he returns with a smaller plate that holds a tiny scoop of hummus, a few small pieces of pita, and ten almonds. This I can eat.

At bedtime, Jeff helps me to and from the commode, squeezes toothpaste onto my toothbrush, replaces the slightly soiled disposable pad on my mattress with a fresh one, and gets me situated in bed. He brings me my medications—low-dose antidepressants and antianxiety pills for sleep, supplements for my immune system, painkillers for the still-open incision. Once I'm settled he climbs into our bed, an arm's length from me. Spike joins him and curls up at the foot of the bed. Jeff turns out the lamp on the bedside table, and the total darkness is surprising. So too is the quiet. There are no humming machines, no footsteps or voices in the distance, no light streaming in from the hallway. There is only peace.

And then, it happens. The repetitious wheezing noise of Spike's favorite squeaky toy, her worn and nappy plush bone, disrupts the quiet. This is one of her favorite pranks: wait for lights out, give it thirty seconds or so, and blast us with what we have come to call her "concerts," which have never failed to make us laugh. But Jeff wants my first night sleeping at home to be without incident, perhaps to convince me that I'll be fine without my usual nursing team, perhaps to convince himself.

"Spike, no!" Jeff scolds, his voice muted, yet harsh. "Bad dog!"

"It's okay," I say. "In fact, it's perfect." And I mean it. To me, this is Spike's way of welcoming me, of accepting me back into the pack. She continues her concert as tears roll down my cheeks. This is the sound of home.

24

AFTER FIFTEEN HOURS OF UNINTERRUPTED SLEEP, I awaken in the same position Jeff arranged me in last night: on my back, head and legs slightly elevated, arms at my sides—the only way I'm comfortable. I look around, confirming that I am indeed home: *my* bedroom, *my* blankets, *my* decorations on the walls. And there, in those photos: *my* baby.

In one, Clare is wrapped in a towel, resting her head against Dede's shoulder. She looks pensive, like a wee soul who fully understands the calamitous circumstances of her birth and the jarring separation from her parents. Yet those knowing eyes are trapped in a tiny physical body that only consciously understands eat-poop-sleep, eat-poop-sleep. And when the knowingness overwhelms, her only means of expression is cry, cry more, keep crying.

This is not how I intended my first months as a new mom to be. I had plans, *big* plans. I was going to breastfeed, make my own baby food with fruits and vegetables from the little organic grocer on 24th Street, maybe even sign up with an eco-friendly cloth diaper service. Becoming pregnant gave me the desire to change, to be a better person for my child.

I don't allow my thoughts to linger on Clare, am not ready to fully grasp our shared sorrow. Hell, I'm still not able to fully grasp, or even look at, the open surgical wound on my belly, which the doctors have said could take months to fully close. How can I possibly expect to look deeper, to the emotional wounds of this experience, the wounds that will still be healing years from now?

"You awake?" Jeff asks, leaning into the room, one hand on the doorknob for balance.

"Yeah," I say. "Can you help me up? I really have to pee."

Jeff brings my walker to the bed, pulls me to sitting, and drapes my fleece robe around my shoulders before easing my arms through their respective sleeves. I work the buttons on the hospital bed to raise the mattress as high as it will go, which allows me to simply lean forward to standing. So far, so good. I make my way across the room and down the hallway toward the living area, pausing every two steps to catch my breath. Val and Bev are sitting on the couch, so I lift a hand in greeting, too winded to form words. Once I'm in the main bathroom, Jeff eases me onto the toilet, pulls me up when I'm finished, and wipes my behind. I turn to the sink to wash my hands and brush my teeth.

"I'm okay now," I say. "I can do this part by myself." Tentatively, Jeff leaves the bathroom, closing the door as he goes.

Too often, my desire to regain independence is trumped by my inability to physically perform basic tasks, but I'm trying. I use one hand to steady myself against the sink while turning on the faucet with the other. Halfway through brushing my teeth, my right slipper feels wet, and I look down to see a small steady stream of water leaking from the vanity. I spit, rinse, and turn off the faucet, then reach down and open the cabinet door under the sink. Rolls of toilet paper are swollen with moisture and there's a puddle surrounding the cleaning products, shampoo bottles, and boxes of tampons. I can neither see the source of the leak nor lower myself enough to pull out the contents of the vanity.

"Jeff?" I call out. The pocket door to the bathroom quickly slides open and there is my husband, a look of expectant dread on his face.

"What is it?" he asks, panic in his voice. This isn't the first time since coming home yesterday that Jeff responded with a level of urgency disproportionate to the situation, as if his reactions are now ruled by an irrational hypervigilance, his psyche unable to grasp that we are no longer in crisis mode. He looks worn, the seams of his steady pragmatism frayed.

"We have a leak," I say, motioning downward with my head while leaning on my walker for support. "Doesn't look too bad, but we may have to call the landlord to get it fixed." Jeff's expression relaxes and he squats down in front of the open cabinet door.

"Let's have a look," he says, pulling out soggy toilet paper rolls and tossing them in the trash can. I watch as Jeff clears out the contents of the vanity. It feels good, almost comforting, to focus on a small challenge that is completely unrelated to my health and well-being..

"Ah, there it is," says Jeff. "Looks like I just need to tighten it." He stands and heads toward the kitchen, where he keeps a small inventory of tools. Leaning toward the open vanity, I see a small rusty wing nut attached to a valve, which is dripping. My husband is no handyman, but this looks pretty straightforward. Jeff returns, pliers in hand, and squats down, his upper body disappearing as he leans into the vanity.

"Goddammit!" he says.

"What is it?"

"Fuck!"

"What!"

"I broke the damn nut off!"

The water continues to leak at the same slow pace, but clearly we need the assistance of a plumber now. No big deal, certainly nothing our landlord can't or won't handle for us. But Jeff rocks back from his heels to sitting, wraps his arms around his shins, and drops his head to his knees. He says nothing, but his shoulders pump up and down, followed by loud gut-wrenching sobs, the likes of which I've never heard come from him.

"It's okay, honey," I say. "I'm okay. Everything's fine now."

His wailing continues, a torrent of pent-up fear and angst and doubt and sorrow. Gripping my walker, I watch my husband surrender to the psychic burden he has carried for more than six weeks. I'm unable to slide down the bathroom wall and sit by his side, unable to bend down enough to wrap him in my arms. I simply look on from above, tears rolling down my cheeks. But just as I cannot let my gaze linger on photographs of Clare, still living four hundred miles away, I'm incapable of looking directly at the full impact of my illness—on myself, on my baby, on Jeff. I pivot my walker and leave.

"I think he needs you," I say to Bev, who's standing right outside the bathroom door. I shuffle past her, making my way to the lift chair, where Val helps me get settled. I overhear fragments of Bev's soothing words and picture her rubbing Jeff's back, as if he's still that young boy she comforted when he fell from his Stingray bike or got knocked over by the family's Great Dane. Val and I say nothing, both eavesdropping on Jeff's posttraumatic heartache, the final dismantling of his stoic armor.

Minutes pass, and Val's expression shifts to one of feigned annoyance. "Oh, get over it already," she says softly, so only the two of us can hear. Our hands instantly fly to our mouths to quell irrepressible snorts of sophomoric amusement.

"You're bad," I say.

"You were thinking the same thing," she replies.

"Maybe, maybe not."

We continue in this vein, turning the sorrow of a man we both dearly love into sound bites of juvenile banter. Humor, Val has learned and I am learning, is at the heart of healing. It can inject a dose of levity to an otherwise disheartening scenario—thoughts of a long recovery for me, or of no recovery for Val. Over the years, I've watched my sister-in-law's comedic outlook grow in proportion to her worsening MS symptoms, a resignation not to the tragedy of her life, but to the absurdity of it.

Half an hour after his breakdown began, Jeff emerges from the bathroom, eyes red, but no longer crying. He offers Val and me a weak smile and sits beside his sister on the couch. Bev goes to the kitchen to make scrambled eggs, toast, and hot tea. After breakfast and a call to the landlord about the bathroom leak, the four of us sit in the living room making plans for the day. Jeff wants to run a few errands. Val wants to read. I want to do nothing at all.

"How about we wash your hair, Lauren?" Bev says. Jeff and Val look at each other, eyes wide.

"What's wrong with my hair?" I ask, knowing full well how slick with oil it is.

"Nothing," says Jeff. "Other than the fact that you look like you've been raised in the wilderness by wolves."

It's true. Except for one shampooing in the hospital, the last time I washed my hair was two days before Clare's birth, as I prepared for dinner at a high-end restaurant with Jeff and his friend Ric, who was in town on business. I wore my crushed velvet maternity mini-dress, high heels, and the pearls Jeff gave me as a wedding gift. I reveled in Ric's unabashed flirting, ignoring the fact that he was gay. For a woman who was eight months pregnant, I looked damn fine and I knew it. But now my jaundiced skin has turned from a Bart Simpson yellow to a George Hamilton bronze. I smell of a body in decay or detox or both. And my hair is matted in no particular pattern all over my head.

"So you don't like the Wolf Girl look?" I ask.

"It's not your best," Val says.

"Can we do it tomorrow?" I ask.

Right now, the thought of having to stand at the sink for ten minutes seems impossible, and it's difficult for me to describe the sudden depletion of my stamina. It's as if there are distinct units of energy that are burned off with every physical action I perform. If a normally functioning person has a thousand energy units to use in a single day, I used to have fifteen hundred, some days two thousand. Yet in this post-ICU world, I feel as if I have ten units of energy for an entire day. A journey down the hallway with my walker costs me two, four for the round-trip. An hour awake and sitting upright is another unit. Reading for thirty minutes, one more. I must monitor the use of my units carefully, for when they're depleted, so too am I. There's no going into overdrive, no drawing on adrenaline reserves. Those were exhausted in the hospital.

"You could sit in the wheelchair and we could back you up to the shower," Val suggests.

"That might work," I say, willing to give it a try.

"If you two want to run errands, I can wash Wa's hair while you're gone," Val says to Jeff and Bev.

"You sure you can handle that?" Jeff asks.

"How hard can it be?" Val says.

"You really don't like the Wolf Girl look, do you?" I say to Val, already knowing the answer.

"Don't make me answer that, Wa," she replies, a wicked smile on her face.

"Okay," Jeff says. "We'll be fast. Just need a few groceries, and I might make a couple other stops."

I can see the relief on my husband's face, the chance to go into the real world with his mother, to walk among the normal people. Before leaving, he helps me transfer from my lift chair to the wheelchair. At the door, he turns back to us.

"You're sure you'll be okay?"

"Go!" Val and I shout in unison. The front door closes and I let out a deep sigh. A break from Jeff's emotional frailty is a welcome gift.

"He's a bit of a basket case," Val says.

"No kidding."

"Well, let's do this."

Val backs my wheelchair into the bathroom and up against the tub. My head is still more than a foot from the edge, and we realize we've grossly miscalculated the ease of washing my hair this way.

"Maybe the kitchen sink? You could stay in the chair and lean forward," Val says. She pushes me out of the bathroom and into the kitchen. No luck. The sink is too high and again the wheels restrict our access.

"This is stupid," I say. "I'll just stand and you can work fast." Val agrees. She slides her forearms under my armpits to give me a boost up. We take the "on three" approach, but when we hit three my bottom remains on the vinyl seat of the wheelchair. We both laugh.

"One more try," she says. But again we reach three to no avail, and again we laugh. By our fourth failed attempt, neither Val nor I are laughing. I don't have the strength to push out of the chair, and she doesn't have the strength to pull me up from it. She wheels me back to the living room, then flops on the couch. Her energy units seem depleted as well.

"We're pathetic," I say.

"We'll never hear the end of it from my brother."

And so we sit and talk like old college friends at a ten-year reunion, our discussion wandering from topic to topic, but then lingering on our newly discovered alliance: what it's like to have the entire family worried about you, to be the focal point of so much angst and concern, and what it's like to have a strong powerful body taken away through illness. Val and I now have a bond that supersedes that of being sisters-in-law. We have the bond of lost health.

An hour passes, and my bladder feels the need for relief. "Hate to tell you this, Val, but I've got to pee."

"Okay, we can do this," she says.

But again, we can't. I call Jeff's cell phone.

"What's wrong?" he answers, without so much as a hello. The last thing I want is to panic him, so I simply ask how much longer he thinks he'll be.

"We have one more stop. Do you need me to come home now?" he asks. The hypervigilance has crept back into his voice. "Oh no, no," I say. "We're fine. I was just curious." Jeff and I say goodbye.

"I'll just hold it," I tell Val, and we continue talking. Soon, I feel a different sensation within my body.

"Oh shit," I say.

"What?"

"I have to poop."

Val snickers, covers her mouth, snickers some more. Again, she tries to help me stand, and again, both of us lack the strength to get me out of this wheelchair. I dial Jeff's cell number and tell him the truth. He says he'll be right there, so I hang up and will my bowels to hold tight. Val drops her head and slowly shakes it back and forth.

"He'll never leave me with you again," she says, and we both start to laugh, causing me to wet myself, which makes us laugh even harder.

Sometimes, humor is all we have.

25

AFTER THE OVEREXERTION OF YESTERDAY, I went to bed early—my hair still oily and matted—and slept a solid fourteen hours. Today, I'm determined to let someone wash my hair before I deplete my daily allowance of energy units. Grasping the bar over my head, I hoist myself up, drop my legs off the side of the bed, and take hold of my walker. Putting on a robe or nightgown seems like too much effort, so I shuffle toward the living area wearing nothing but my slippers and the large bandage taped loosely over my lower abdomen. Jeff, Val, and Bev hear me coming down the hallway and call out their hellos.

"She lives!" Val says.

"Look who finally woke up," Bev adds.

"Morning, hon," Jeff calls out.

I come into their line of vision, and all three of them erupt in laughter over my nakedness and apparent lack of embarrassment. I stop and take a few labored breaths.

"Wolf Girl has arrived," I say, causing more hilarity.

If I could catch my breath I would laugh too. The absurdity of how I must look to them—hunched over my walker, bronze greasy skin, unkempt hair, emaciated breasts, no pubic hair, and ubiquitous bruises—is not lost on me. I saw my naked body as I passed the mirrored closet doors in the bedroom. I look like a cadaver, something straight out of *Tales from the Crypt*. But unlike times in the past, when the discovery of a few cellulite dimples on my butt or the start of a paunch on my belly would send me reeling all the way to the gym, my body is so vastly altered from my mind's perception of what I'm supposed to look like that I find the changes more amusing than disturbing. Preeclampsia has hurled me from the uppermost rung of Maslow's hierarchy of needs—the self-actualization level, focusing on identity and purpose—down to the lowest rung, the one focused on the most basic physiological needs: food, water, excretion, sleep. That about sums up the entirety of my schedule these days: eat-drink-poop-nap, eat-drink-poop-nap. It's as if Clare and I are neck and neck in the race to develop, right down to our use of diapers, or in my case, disposable under-pads.

"Does anyone want to wash my hair?" I ask.

"Yes!" they all yell in unison. More laughter.

"Okay, let's get it over with before I run out of energy," I say.

My mother-in-law meets me at the kitchen sink and Jeff runs to the bathroom for shampoo. I lean forward and Bev washes my hair while Val gives me a sponge bath. Jeff brings a fresh nightgown from the bedroom and slips it over my head. He then helps me get settled in my lift chair for a breakfast of tea and toast and banana slices.

Within an hour of being bathed, I'm greasy again. We all marvel at how quickly I went from clean and dry to slick with oil. With my liver and kidneys still convalescing, my skin and scalp provide the fastest route for the toxic gunk to exit my body. Brimming with curiosity, Jeff wipes my forehead with a white washcloth, and when he pulls it away we both say *Ewww* because it's now stained yellow. He retrieves a fresh washcloth from the bathroom and repeats his experiment, this time on one of my arms. Again, the washcloth comes away with a yellow stain.

"Looks like Wolf Girl is here to stay," he says. "At least for the time being."

"And Wolf Girl is exhausted," I say. With Jeff's help I return to the bedroom and sleep for three more hours.

"Katherine's here," Jeff says, leaning into the bedroom. "You up for a little visit?"

"Sure," I tell Jeff.

I've not yet agreed to have visitors outside of my inner circle of friends and family who helped in the hospital. Any visit, even a brief one, requires more energy than I can afford. I've averaged twenty hours of sleep a day since coming home and still I'm exhausted after the simplest activities. When Jeff poked his head in the bedroom on my first day home to tell me that a neighbor was here and wanted to say hello, I made him send her away. His expression told me he thought I was being unreasonable, and I could hear the embarrassment in his voice when he went to the front door, twenty feet from the bedroom, and apologetically told her we'd have to do it another day. Since then, he's played the role of gatekeeper, diplomatically telling friends who call not to come, that he'll be in touch when I'm ready to have visitors.

But Katherine is different. We've lived across the street from her for three years, stopping to chat when we passed her condo on our way to Dolores Park with Spike and allowing our respective dogs a few minutes of butt sniffing and wrestling in her front yard. Recently, I learned of her kindness while I was in the hospital, how she dropped off pillows and blankets when our home was packed with out-of-town family members, and how she hosted a blood drive at the private school she owns when she heard the local supplies were running low.

During our five-minute visit, I come to better understand the motivation behind Katherine's generosity and concern during my hospitalization.

"I had preeclampsia too," she says. "I almost lost Mary Katherine when she came two months early."

When Katherine leaves, Jeff sits on the edge of my bed and updates me on the logistics of integrating Clare back into our lives. He's been on the phone with Tim and Dede, and they understand that we need more time to establish my routine with home-care nurses and physical therapists before our baby comes home to live with us. They were less understanding, Jeff tells me, about his desire to have them fly up from Orange County with Clare for a day so Bev and Val can meet our baby before they go home. He believes it'll be a long time before we're able to travel to Michigan, given my rehabilitation needs, so he's eager, borderline desperate, to have her brought to San Francisco for a quick visit while his mother and sister are still here.

But Tim declined, Jeff tells me, reminding him that Dede has three small children to care for in addition to our baby. And since Tim is self-employed, if he doesn't work he doesn't get paid, and he's already lost a considerable amount of work time with his trips to be with me in the hospital. As Jeff recounts these conversations for me, I can hear the disappointment in his voice. Not anger, but sadness and exhaustion and resignation.

"You need a nature break, Jeff," I say. "A few days, maybe even a week, away somewhere. Yosemite, or someplace like that."

Ever since I've known him, Jeff's trips to nature have always proved to be the perfect antidote for whatever ails him. I've always supported, even encouraged, his weekend backpacking trips because I knew he'd return rejuvenated. Gone would be whatever dark cloud hung over his head before he left, and in its place an aura of fresh ideas, renewed possibilities, and excitement for the future.

"Well, that's not going to happen," he says, glumly.

"Why not? You just told me we have almost two weeks before Clare comes home. Mom could fly out and babysit me, and you could go somewhere and get rejuvenated."

"I couldn't do that."

Even as he says the words, I sense it's a knee-jerk reaction, one I've seen before with him, a blatant disregard for his own needs because he feels it wouldn't be right. But after four years with him, I know the best strategy for responding.

"Let's face it," I say. "You and the nanny Pam hired for us are going to have to do all the baby care for a while. You need to be refreshed for Clare's sake. You need to do this for *her*."

I can see his mind at work, the mental wrestling match between his usual perspective that to do something for himself would be selfish and this new perspective that revitalization is a critical aspect of his paternal obligation to Clare.

"It *would* be good for me, wouldn't it?" he says. A little smile crosses his face, and it appears his mind is wandering off to one of the beautiful gorges he's hiked in the past.

He needs this. *I* need this. I need my husband back, the one whose confidence and joy are authentic, whose belief that good things lie ahead isn't faked. Ever since becoming conscious—and sane—I've seen few expressions of honest pleasure on Jeff's face, as if his body and mind were perpetually on alert for the next surprise attack, even after we came home. It reminds me of the time we were walking down 24th Street with Spike off-leash and a passing Doberman pinscher lunged for her, its teeth coming within inches of her jugular before the owner yanked back hard on its leash. Spike had sensed she was toast and instead of running, she lay down in defeat, baring her neck for her attacker. The owner apologized profusely and we walked on, but Spike was noticeably traumatized for the next half a mile, her gait awkward, her head bent low, and her interest in cats and scents and other canine pleasures nonexistent. Finally, at the top of the hill leading to our home, she shook her body hard and furiously, as if she'd just emerged from a lake, heavy with excess water. She shook and shook until the trauma of the Doberman pinscher encounter was cast from her body and her psyche. Only then did she return to normal, pouncing toward a squirrel and then bounding back toward Jeff and me for approval, her aren't-I-a-clever-dog smile restored, her joy palpable.

Jeff needs a good shake. He needs to immerse himself in fresh air and mountaintops and the smell of wild grasses, and shake all the heartache and fear and shock of the last two months from his soul.

"Katherine said you could use her place in Jackson Hole if you want."

"Huh."

"Lots of great hiking there. And I think it was a sincere offer on her part."

"You know, the idea of pissing off a mountaintop does hold appeal," he says, a look of genuine enthusiasm on his face. "Okay, let's do it."

Over the next several days, I work on the details of Jeff's trip, buying his airline ticket, helping him figure out what to pack. I like focusing on someone else's needs, and it feels good to help my husband for a change. Katherine stops by to drop off keys to her condo in Wyoming, as well as the keys to a minivan she keeps parked at the airport—an unexpected bonus. Then she stays with me while Jeff drives Val and Bev to the airport for their return to Michigan.

The next afternoon, Jeff leaves for the airport to catch his flight, which is scheduled to depart shortly before Mom's arrives. With plenty of emergency numbers and the phone by my side, I'm comfortable being left alone for several hours. In fact, I'm thrilled. This is what independence feels like.

Tucked snugly into the hospital bed, I read for a short time before deciding to venture into the guest bedroom. Using my walker, I move across the floor in four-inch increments, out of the master bedroom, through the next doorway, and toward the guest bed, passing the empty crib as I go. I make it to my destination, pivot, and lower myself to sitting. Exhausted, I'm no longer sure why I wanted to come in here.

The heel of my foot brushes against something under the bed and it makes a small rustling sound. Curious, I reach down with my left arm, my right hand grasping the walker for support, my gaze fixed on the far wall to keep the queasiness at bay. My fingers grope the carpet, tug at something, then get it firmly in their grip. Hauling myself upright again, I stare in disbelief. Roses. A bouquet of dead roses.

As I set the flowers in my lap, a few crisp petals fall to the floor. My vision blurs with tears and I'm catapulted back in time. Jeff. Standing in that doorway. Holding these roses. The details of that day flood my senses in a real-time déjà vu: the feigned calm of the doctors and nurses, the panic in my husband's eyes, and the lifeless form of my baby as she was pulled from my womb. The words I spoke as they hustled Clare from the operating room to the neonatal ICU minutes after her birth ring in my head. *Stay with the baby, honey. I'll be fine.*

I smile through tears at that one. At how dead wrong I was.

Jeff's decision to leave work in the middle of back-to-back meetings that afternoon haunts me, his sudden impulse to bring me roses—*these* roses. He'll call it serendipity, but I call it synchronicity, perhaps divine intervention.

Continuing to stare at the parched bouquet, I can't tell if I'm crying with grief for what was lost or gratitude for what wasn't. Before I can determine which it is, a new emotion floods me: guilt. Guilt for the physical warning signs that now seem so obvious, signs to which I might have paid more attention had I not been so naïve about childbirth, so smug about my health. I'd made it thirty-seven years without any major medical crises, so why, I'd thought, should I even consider the possibility that something might go wrong with *my* pregnancy?

"Pregnancy karma will catch up with you," one of my mom-friends had jokingly said to me during my first trimester when I bragged about having an easy time of it. "If you have a lot of morning sickness early on, you'll have a peaceful third trimester. But if your first trimester is a breeze, your last few months will be crappy."

Later, I remembered her tongue-in-cheek wisdom when minor yet aggravating symptoms started occurring in my eighth month: bloating and gas, puffy club-like feet that forced me to wear slippers to my baby shower, legs and ankles that thickened disproportionately to the rest of my girth, and a ubiquitous fatigue. I assumed these were all normal. After all, pregnancy complications happened to other people, not to me.

My capacity for denial knew no bounds. As Jeff, Spike, and I drove home from a weekend getaway in Mendocino four days before Clare's birth, I suddenly experienced severe jolts of pain in the upper right side of my abdomen. I tilted the passenger seat all the way back and tried lying flat, then on my side, then on my other side, but the cramping continued.

"Do you think something's wrong?" Jeff asked.

"No. It's probably just gas," I replied. "Or maybe I need to eat something."

We pulled into the next Taco Bell, which had become a routine craving of mine over the past eight months. Jeff ordered my usual—Meal Deal #3 with crunchy shells, beans instead of meat, extra cheese, and a Pepsi—while I sat in a booth with my arms wrapped around my belly trying to hug the pain away. A suspicion that something might be wrong crept into my mind, but I ignored it. *If I deny the thought, it can't come true.*

Whether it was the food or the break from driving or something else altogether, the pain subsided after I ate, and both Jeff and I assumed the incident was inconsequential. Naïveté prevailed. The next day's prenatal checkup showed nothing out of the ordinary: normal blood pressure, no protein in my urine. I didn't bother mentioning the abdominal issue to my doctor.

At lunchtime three days later, I had another urge for Taco Bell, but the effort to shower, dress, and drive seemed like too much, even for Meal Deal #3. Instead, I shuffled to the kitchen in my pajamas and ate a few crackers with cheese, then shuffled back down the hallway for another nap. The master bedroom was awash in midday sunlight from windows on three walls, so I opted for the small guest bedroom with only one window, a twin bed, and the desk I'd used for consulting work during the first half of my pregnancy. I crawled into bed, *this* bed, and pulled the covers around me. Spike jumped up and wedged her forty-five-pound body between the wall and my legs. At ten after two, I was startled from sleep by the banging of the security gate, followed by the sound of a key in the front door and Jeff's voice. *Hello?* And then my husband, roses in hand, appeared in the doorway a full six hours before he was expected home. During my entire pregnancy, he'd never left work to check on me. Called, yes. Come in person, no. Later, after the doctor told us that Clare was in trouble and needed to be delivered immediately, I asked Jeff why he'd decided to come home so early; why not wait until the end of the day to bring me those roses?

"I was sitting in a meeting and Margaret was saying something, but all I could hear was the voice of Charlie Brown's teacher: *Wanh, wanh, wanh, wanh, wanh,*" he said, mimicking the elusive cartoon character's voice. "It wasn't that I sensed something was wrong. It was more like a sudden inexplicable urge to bring you flowers, to remind you—*us*—to stop and smell the roses."

"Really?"

"Yeah. Strange, huh?"

My pregnancy had consisted of 246 days during which Jeff could've brought me roses. Why *that* day?

I make my way back to the master bedroom, pausing at the nightstand to pull my journal from the top drawer. It has been months since I wrote and I have difficulty gripping a pen, but the desire to record my thoughts supersedes the challenges of doing so. Once resettled in the hospital bed, I randomly flip the journal open to an entry dated December 30, 1999. I'd recently begun my seventh month of pregnancy and we were visiting

Jeff's family in Michigan for the holidays. Late-night insomnia had sent me to the atrium to reflect, Bev's many plants and the gentle tinkling of the water fountain in the corner providing a meditative backdrop. *Over the past couple months,* I had written, *I've been in awe at how well my life, and Jeff's and my life together, is going. Love, prosperity, joy, Clare—lots of goodness happening. At times, I wonder if the other shoe will drop—the sudden death of Jeff or some other calamity.*

Whoa. Had I ignored more than the physical signs? Were there intuitive signs as well? If the desire to bring me roses was Jeff's subconscious prompt that something was awry, were these inner musings mine? I continue reading page after page, and in the final journal entry before Clare's arrival, the last words I'd written were these: *I LOVE BEING PREGNANT. Thanks, Life.*

I sit, stunned, with the discovery that my final observation before going into a medical tailspin was adulation for that which nearly killed me. And then, another jolt. On the pages that follow, Jeff's handwriting, sloppy and rushed, forms a bullet-pointed account of my failed health.

Coagulation and encephalopathy = indicators of liver failure.
Status One.
Oozing = clot grows.
Stage 4 (coma).

And below that are his questions, written weeks later, their numbering as disjointed as his thinking must've been by then.

(7) Have you ever performed this operation on patients with liver and kidney failure?

(11) What is the penalty for delay if the uterus is infected?

(12) If there is a dispute between the liver team and the OB team about the hysterectomy, how is that mediated?

Reading through page after page of Jeff's questions, I begin to have a few of my own. Like, how did he manage to pull himself through this ordeal, day after day, hour after hour? What must it have been like for him, the guy who was ambivalent about having children in the first place, to consider the real possibility of becoming both a father and a widower in the same week? Did he ever think back on that day and wonder about the likely outcome had he *not* followed his instinct to bring me flowers? And why on earth did he take notes in my journal? To my knowledge, he'd never breached our agreement to allow one another our private thoughts on paper. I'm not upset by this discovery. Just perplexed. This is the first of many gaps in a story I have yet to fully understand.

26

By the second day of Mom's visit, we've established a nice routine. I sleep about fourteen hours each night and another three to four during the day. During my daytime naps, Mom reads or pays my bills or organizes our home more than it already is. Her latest project—alphabetizing the spices in our kitchen cupboard—is, I suspect, retribution for my unmerciful teasing during a visit years ago when I discovered her spice drawer with its orderly Basil through Vanilla Bean arrangement. For fun, I covertly switched her Chili Powder with her Thyme to see how long it would take her to figure it out. I received an accusatory e-mail from her the day after I left Boulder.

When I'm awake, Mom makes me small plates of food, simple stuff like her buttery mashed potatoes or tuna salad, both childhood favorites. Every morning I crave a poached egg, which she's relearned how to make for me. She cajoles me into doing my deep-breathing exercises with the little contraption they gave me at the hospital. I'm still unable to take a full breath, but my lung capacity is slowly improving. And at night, when I'm tucked into a comfortable position at bedtime, she reads to me from the same book Jeff read to me in the hospital. I find my mother's voice as enchanting as it was when I was a young girl and she read to my brother and sisters and me from our seemingly massive set of storybooks. When it was my turn to pick the story, I always chose *Teeny-Tiny* or *How Brer Rabbit Met Brer Tar Baby* because I loved Mom's impersonations of the characters.

On our third day together, I lie naked on the portable massage table I bought a year ago, remembering the last time I was on it: my thirty-eighth birthday, three months earlier, on an overcast Saturday. Jeff woke me that morning holding a champagne glass of orange juice and the first of several birthday gifts—a chrome bathtub tray. He led me to the living room, where he had a fire burning and candles lit. Set up by the fireplace was the massage table, with extra pillows to accommodate my bulging belly. After gently rubbing me with aromatherapy oils, Jeff wrapped me in my fluffy floor-length robe, sat me on the couch, and laid out a feast of fresh bagels, lox, tomatoes, and cream cheese on the coffee table. Next came a hot bubble bath. As I settled my seven-months-pregnant body into the tub, Jeff poured more orange juice into my glass and set a little plate of rich dark chocolates on my new tray. When the bathwater cooled, he boiled more on the stove, our water heater never having been quite robust enough to heat the amount needed for a long and satisfying soak. After my bath, we went back to the bedroom and made love, only later discovering that my friend Carrie had stopped by unexpectedly and left a gift at the front door. The doorbell never rang, so Jeff and I assumed the commotion within had acted as a do-not-disturb sign.

Today, it's not Jeff who's giving me a massage, but Dusa. It took a team effort by her and Mom to get me onto the table and on my back, pillows padding my knees and feet and neck. This is Dusa's third in-home appointment with me, and the first time she's incorporating massage techniques into the treatment. Normally, she doesn't make house calls, but she's bending the rules for me, at least until I'm well enough to leave my home and come to her office. I don't understand all the facets of her work, but as she strokes my arms and legs in long slow motions, I sense it is healing me on levels I can't comprehend. Spike seems to sense this too. She sits near the massage table watching every move, like an eager assistant waiting for her next task assignment.

Soon, the massaging stops and Dusa pulls the lightweight blanket up over my body. A minute or two passes and I open my eyes to see her doing that weird little thing with her hands, as she did when I was in the ICU. Her eyes are closed and her hands move in sweeping, then circular, motions up and down my body, but always about five inches above it.

"What *is* that you're doing?" I ask. She opens her eyes and smiles at me.

"I'm working on repairing the holes in your energy field," she says.

"Huh?"

"Imagine that you have an energetic casing around your body. During trauma, it's not unusual for holes to appear in it, so I'm smoothing them away to strengthen your energy field."

"Do I have a lot of holes?" I ask, curious, standing on the border between skepticism and belief.

"Quite a few," she says, continuing to move her hands over these holes I can't see. "But you've come a long way since the hospital."

"That bad, huh?"

"I remember the day we met. Your energy field looked like land mines had erupted everywhere. I honestly didn't know where to begin."

"Well, whatever you did, it seemed to help. Even my stepdad, the world's biggest skeptic, said that he saw a huge difference in me after you left."

"Everyone there—you, your husband, your parents—*every-one* was traumatized by your illness, Lauren. I tried to give them confidence in your body's ability to heal."

"I think it worked," I say.

I close my eyes and allow Dusa to continue her work in silence. When she's finished, she tells me to relax on the table a few more minutes. Then I hear her addressing Spike.

"You've been through a lot, too, haven't you?" she says. "How about we do a little energy work on you while your mama rests?"

I turn my head to the left and watch as Dusa kneels next to Spike and places her hands on my dog's body, shifting position every thirty seconds or so. Spike doesn't flinch. She sits, calm and steady, for a full ten-minute treatment, soaking in what Dusa has to offer.

Afterward, I move to the hospital bed for a nap. When I awaken, I eat a small lunch of raw almonds, hummus and pita, and organic ginger ale. I ask Mom to help me get in the shower, my first since the day before Clare's birth. I'm nervous about the spray of water on my surgical wound, though it has closed a bit more each day. The incision now looks like the top of a Ziploc bag that is partially unsealed at one end. About two inches long, it no longer needs to be packed with gauze. A five-inch by five-inch bandage is sufficient to keep dust or other contaminants from causing infection.

Mom places our new portable shower chair on top of the bath mat in the tub. I join her in the tiny bathroom so she can lift my legs, one at a time, over the side of the tub. My left hand holds the handle on the sliding shower door while my right hand clenches a wad of the shirt on Mom's back. We are laughing at how ridiculous we must look: she, bent over like a rag doll, and me, a mass of dead weight that she must somehow transport into the tub. Once in, I sit on the chair and catch my breath as Mom pulls the handheld showerhead from its wall mount and adjusts the water temperature. She gives me a small dry towel to cover my incision and hands me the shower wand. I start with my feet to test the force of the spray on my skin. So far so good. I move up my legs and again am okay with the water pressure. Finally, I move the shower wand up to my arms, shoulders, face, and back. The water feels glorious, the temperature a perfect lukewarm. For a while, I simply sit with the water running over my head and down my back. My balance is still precarious, so Mom waits on the other side of the shower door and hands me the soap, the shampoo, the conditioner as needed. When I'm finished, she hands me a bath towel and I dry myself while seated. Again, we go through the exhausting process of getting each of my legs over the tub's wall. I comb my hair and brush my teeth, then put on a fresh nightgown and robe. I sit in my wheelchair while Mom dries my hair for me, and we marvel at its beautiful new auburn color.

The next morning, Pam arrives unexpectedly with her husband and twin three-year-olds in tow. All four of them are wearing silly headbands with bunny ears or oversized flower petals in bright colors.

"Happy Easter!" they yell, walking into the living room.

"Don't worry," says Pam, "we're just passing through on our way to my dad's house, but Jay really wanted to stop and say hi."

It's a real treat to see my friends. Years ago, I was maid of honor at their wedding, and now, to see them as a family gives me hope. It makes me want to have Clare and Jeff back home, and for the three of us, and Spike, to start our life together as a family. After they leave, I'm energized.

"Can we go to the garage?" I ask Mom. Her expression becomes one of utter disbelief, with good reason. There are two ways to get to the garage and both involve fifteen steps. So far, I've managed to navigate only one step—the one from the front door to the external security gate—to let the visiting nurses in. And I achieved that only by clinging to the doorknob to pull myself back up the step.

"Why on earth do you want to go to the garage?" Mom asks.

"I want to see what we have, what we need. I just want to look around. *Please?*"

"How the hell are we going to get you back up the stairs once we get you down there?" she says. It is more a statement than a question.

"I'll be fine. Promise." As I say these words, I genuinely believe them. My daily ration of energy units seems to be increasing, I tell her. Today, I feel like I've been given thirty. And I really want to do a mundane task, something normal like taking stock of our paper towels and toilet paper. Mom acquiesces but insists on going down the carpeted steps ahead of me. My quadriceps are among the weakest parts of my body, so any movement requiring me to bend my legs is a challenge. Slowly, gingerly, I work my way down each stair backward, clinging with both hands to the handrail, the same way I descended staircases for days after running my first marathon, when my body ached and my quads were shot. I can feel Mom's hands lightly positioned on my butt should I slip, and again we find ourselves laughing at the absurdity of this scene. Halfway down the staircase, Spike skirts past us, her tail wagging. No doubt she believes we're headed for the car, despite the fact that I haven't said her favorite word, *Wannagoforaride.*

We make it to the bottom and Mom opens the door to the garage. Holding my arm, she walks me over to Jeff's old recliner, banished after Spike chewed the corner off its attached footrest. I sink into the soft leather and take in my surroundings, a queen inspecting her kingdom. The garage has room for four cars in two tight rows, but we house only one of our two SUVs there. The rest of the space is taken up by eight bulky warehouse shelving units crammed with suitcases and garment bags, coolers and camping gear, Christmas decorations and party supplies. Excess furniture is shoved haphazardly in a corner: the desk and filing cabinets from my office-turned-nursery, the living room reading chair, a table from the hallway. More recently acquired smaller items crowd the tops of furniture and storage bins: empty casserole dishes belonging to friends and neighbors who fed my visiting family members, extra bags of fertilizer from the welcome-home gardening project, the unused breast pump handed down from Pam. Gone is the organization I worked so hard to perfect during the nesting phase of my pregnancy, and in its place is messiness and disarray. And two things my mother and I both abhor are messiness and disarray.

"Well," she says, "where do we begin?"

For the next hour, Mom straightens and sorts, dusts and disposes. I supervise from my recliner, thrilled to see structure restored. Before leaving the garage, I point out several things we need to bring upstairs with us: a box of tissues for my bedroom, dish detergent, toilet paper, a few dirty towels that need laundering. Mom pulls me up from the chair and walks me to the doorway. I turn back and watch her load her arms with all the items.

"Want some help?" I ask. We both burst out laughing. With a show of drama, she drops everything on the table and walks over to me, pulling something from her back pocket. It's my checkbook, inadvertently left in the car after an errand she ran the other day.

"Here!" she says, stuffing the checkbook into the pocket of my robe. "Make yourself useful."

She returns to her pile of goods, scoops them up again, and joins me at the foot of the stairs. I grab the handrail and yank myself upward, straining. But nothing happens. I will my right leg to bend and lift, but it won't budge.

"Thirty energy units, eh?" Mom says.

"Okay, I can do this," I say. But again my efforts at upward mobility are futile.

"Okay, I *can't* do this," I say.

Mom drops her cargo in the corner and leans in, lifting my right leg onto the first step. Then she gets behind me and, on three, shoves me from my butt up onto the first step. She's exhausted, as am I. We make jokes about Jeff coming home tomorrow night to find me stranded in the garage. Mom sits on the stairs to catch her breath and think through our dilemma.

"I've got an idea," she says. "Try sitting on the stairs like this and use your arms to push yourself up a step. They're a lot stronger than your legs." She stands and helps me lower myself to sitting. I push up with my arms and miraculously my body moves to the next level. I drag my feet up to the next step as well.

"Thank god," I say. "I really didn't want to sleep in the garage." I repeat this pattern a dozen times until my butt rests on the floor of the living room. Mom pulls me up to standing and assists me as I wobble toward the bedroom to lie down.

"I can do it, indeed," she says, a big smirk on her face.

"Bite me!" I reply, and we both crack up. Clearly, laughter requires no energy units.

After dinner, Jeff calls from Wyoming and I can hear the renewal in his voice. He tells me about the hikes he does each day: long ones, eight to ten miles, seeing mountain goats and bighorn sheep and buffalo. Today, he tells me, he had to stop the car on his way to the trailhead and wait ten minutes for a moose to get out of the road. He hikes until his thighs burn and his feet throb. I suspect he hikes to remember who he is and to forget what happened. In the evenings, he goes into town for steak and baked potatoes. He makes no effort to interact with others save for the occasional lifting of an empty beer bottle, indicating *Another, please.*

When my energy wanes, Jeff and I know it's time to say good night. In the week following my hospital discharge, we discovered that if I stay up past eight, I fall apart emotionally. "Eight p.m." has become a euphemism for the time I hit the wall, the time at which I begin to cry for no apparent reason if I'm not safely tucked in bed for the night. It's as if a switch is suddenly and inexplicably thrown, opening the floodgates to my subconscious trauma. A few nights ago, I even laughed while crying because it seemed so absurd that one minute I could be joyfully holding court from my lift chair with several friends and then crying five minutes after their departure at half past eight. "I know, I know," I said through tears as Jeff escorted me to the bedroom after they left.

Before hanging up, Jeff and I say our *I love you's*, and we speak the words as authentically as the day we wed. Nearly losing one another has buffed the complacency off our relationship, and my connection to Jeff feels as clear and conscious and cherished as it was in those early months when we planned our future together, seeing only good things ahead.

"He sounds good," I tell Mom.

"He needed this," she says.

"Amen."

"Bedtime," says Mom. "Want to try sleeping in your real bed for a change?"

Instantly, I shift from happy for Jeff to nervous for me. My real bed doesn't have buttons to adjust the elevation of my legs and back. It doesn't have a triangular bar overhead that I can use to maneuver myself into a comfortable position or to get out of bed if I have to pee. It doesn't have air cushioning so soft it feels like floating in a pool. But I know I can't sleep in the hospital bed forever.

"Okay. I'll give it a try."

I rise from my lift chair all by myself and lean on the walker to regain my balance. Leaving the walker behind, I make my way down the hallway, using the wall to steady myself, the same way I saw Val do it. I brush my teeth and use the commode, then walk to my side of the bed. Mom pulls back the covers and steps away. Tentatively, I sit on the mattress and immediately notice how stony it feels against my bruised bottom. Mom supports my shoulders and head as I lower myself to a prone position. The mattress feels surprisingly hard against my body, as if I'm lying on cinder blocks covered with fabric. I suck in air through clenched teeth as the skin on my back screams from this new and unpleasant sensation.

"You okay?" Mom asks.

"No, but let's give it another minute and see if my body relaxes at all."

Remarkably, it does, so my mother pads me with pillows, gently maneuvering one under my creaky knees, one under each bruised arm, an extra one under my head. She takes one of the stiff pillows and wedges it between the mattress and bed frame at the end of the bed to keep my feet in an upright flexed position. Until they regain their strength, I'm still at risk for foot drop—the tops of my feet weakening during extended periods of sleep, resulting in dragging of the foot and toes. Now that I'm snugly supported with pillows, Mom pulls the blanket over my body, tucks it around my shoulders, and makes incremental adjustments to sheets and blankets and pillows at my direction. I'm thirsty, so she elevates my head with one arm while holding a water cup and straw to my mouth with the other. Then she climbs in bed next to me and reads to me, my own bedtime story. The feeling of comfort I have in this moment is sublime.

By the time Mom has finished reading two chapters, my body has completely relaxed into my old bed, its cellular memory of life before illness slowly returning. She climbs from the bed to leave and at the door she turns back toward me, her hand on the light switch.

"Is there anything else you need right now?" she asks.

Is there anything else I need right now? How often have I heard that question throughout my life, from waiters, hotel staff, employees, even my husband? And how often have I reflexively answered, "I'm fine, thanks," without really thinking about the question? Not this time, though. I keep my knee-jerk response in check and take a moment to think about the question, about my needs. Tomorrow, I'll need energy for my in-home physical therapy appointment. Next week, I'll need the nanny to jump in and take charge of Clare's daytime care. In a year or so, I'll need to reevaluate what my future career possibilities are, based on my level of recovery. And in eighteen years, I'll need funds for my daughter's college education—Berkeley, according to Jeff. But right now, my broken body has given me the gift of living in the present, focusing on the basics of survival. My bladder is empty, my tummy is full, my body is comfortable, and my baby and I are alive.

"You know what, Mom? Right now, I have everything I need. In this moment, my life is perfect."

And I mean it.

27

JEFF WALKS IN THE FRONT DOOR, and I immediately recognize the man I knew before our lives were abruptly changed by blood transfusions and surgeries and medical specialists and a baby we have yet to know. He looks rejuvenated, almost jubilant, his back and shoulders more erect than when he left five days ago. Dropping his duffle bag in the corner, he comes to my lift chair and gives me a kiss. His face is stubbly and his shirt still smells of nature, a mix of campfires and trees and perspiration. He hugs Mom, then flops down on the couch to tell us of his adventures in Wyoming. Seeing him so renewed gives me hope for my own resurrection, our resurrection as a family.

"So it was a good trip," I say, already knowing the answer.

"You have no idea," Jeff says. "It felt so good to work out hard and sweat and not have to talk to any doctors—to *anyone*, for that matter."

"So you didn't tell anyone about what happened?" I ask.

If the tables were turned and I were the one going on a retreat to recover my mental well-being, I'd bend the ears of the other people checking in at the airport, the person sitting next to me on the plane, the flight attendant when she drops a napkin and a pack of nuts on my tray table and asks for my drink order. I would spread my grief around without the filter of propriety, parceling it out left and right in hopes of diluting its magnitude in my own life.

"No one," he says. "Until today. I was taking off my boots at the trailhead after my hike and noticed one other hiker at his car, so we struck up a conversation about how beautiful it was on the trail."

"What happened?" Mom asks, walking toward the kitchen to get him a glass of water.

"He asked if I was from around there and when I said no, I suddenly found myself telling him everything, from start to finish. Halfway through my story, he interrupts me, leans into the back of his SUV, and pulls out a couple beers from a cooler. 'Here,' he says, 'I think you need this.' So we sat and talked and drank together. It felt good, actually, to tell the whole story to a complete stranger."

Jeff pauses, as if reflecting. Unable to contain myself anymore, I blurt out my news.

"I stopped using my walker!" I say.

"Really?" he says. "That's fantastic, Lauren!"

"And I walked up the stairs," I add.

"That one?" he asks, pointing to the entranceway with its lone step down to the front door.

"Those stairs!" I say, pointing toward the staircase that leads down to the garage. "All fifteen of them!" I'm beaming with pride as Mom fills in the details of my backward crab walk up the staircase yesterday and my determination to do it again earlier today, this time standing. I made it the whole way, needing help from the visiting physical therapist only on the last three steps from the top.

Mom excuses herself to get ready for bed, her flight home less than twelve hours away. I thank her for coming to babysit me since I'll be deep in sleep when the cab arrives to take her to the airport tomorrow morning.

"You know, hon," Jeff says, "I did a lot of thinking while I was in Wyoming."

"And?"

"We've always said that someday we'd like to move to Boulder. After what we just went through, doesn't it feel like someday is today?"

"You mean move there *now*?"

I am simultaneously thrilled and nervous. It's a big decision, but Jeff and I already have a track record of making our biggest decisions in life—getting married, becoming parents—with the greatest level of spontaneity. At times, we have spent more time and energy deciding which restaurant to eat at than we did making life-altering choices.

"Why not?" he says. "We would wait until you're well enough to leave your San Francisco doctors. And maybe I could telecommute to work, fly back for the important meetings, and do the rest from Boulder." Just as I coaxed Jeff into taking a temporary retreat in the Rockies, now he's coaxing me into taking a permanent one.

"I suppose if it didn't work out we could always move back," I say.

"Exactly!"

"Mom and John could help us out during my recovery. Could we live near them?"

"Absolutely! That's what I was thinking too."

"Maybe my hallucinations about being in Colorado while I was in the hospital were a sign." We both laugh, giddy with the possibilities of a fresh start, a new beginning. A new life.

"How about if I call Matt tomorrow to see if he's cool with me telecommuting," he says. Additional payments from the sale of Jeff's company six months ago are contingent on his staying with the acquiring company for two more years. And we can't afford to walk from those payments, not now, not with a new baby and a long-term recovery for me. Matt's blessing is the first step in making our plans a reality.

Thoughts of a new beginning in Boulder permeate every cell in my body, images of past visits projected into our future, this time with Clare and Spike at our side: walks down 4th Street to Jeff's favorite coffee shop; the beauty of the Flatirons with winter's first dusting of snow; the smell of Mom and John's woodburning fireplace as the four of us read our books, perhaps while Clare naps in a portable crib in the corner of their living room. My senses overwhelmed, I begin to cry. Both Jeff and I look at the clock over the kitchen sink. It's 9:05, long past my bedtime. "Did it again," he says.

Jeff hoists me up from my lift chair and walks with me toward the bedroom, where he helps me with my nighttime routine and tucks me into our bed. I hear him move through the house, turning off lights, locking the French doors to the patio, brushing his teeth in the main bathroom. He returns and climbs under the sheets next to me. The last time we slept in the same bed was fifty-four days ago, when I was pregnant and full of hope for the future. Now, I'm no longer pregnant, but my sense of hope is returning.

Spike hops on the bed from Jeff's side and stretches out near our feet, squeaky toy in mouth. As she serenades us with her evening concert, Jeff turns out the light and lies on his side facing me. We continue to talk about our future life in Boulder. Jeff describes how he'll start biking with my stepdad, and hiking alone. One day, he tells me, he'll go back to school to study philosophy and history. He has shared this dream before, his desire to earn a PhD. Underneath all that business attire and corporate-speak, my husband is a scholar at heart, the pursuit of knowledge more compelling to him than any mergers, product innovations, or year-end results.

I talk of exploring different alternative healing methods to help with my recovery, Boulder being the de facto capital of all things off the beaten path. I describe how I'll learn to do yoga, make more time for meditation, perhaps begin writing in earnest. And someday when I'm strong enough, my legs will pump down 4th Street as I push Clare in the extra-tall purple baby jogger my siblings gave me at my shower in February. We'll meet up with Jeff and John at a coffee shop on Pearl Street at the end of their bike ride. Mom will drive John's minivan downtown to meet all of us, after which she can transport us home in comfort. I fall asleep holding onto these images as tightly as I hold Jeff's hand.

The following morning, Jeff decides to go to work for the first time in eight weeks. I'm now capable of easily moving to and from the front door to let in the physical therapist or the nurse or my kidney doctor-neighbor, who has offered to make in-home checkups. My husband looks triumphant, ready for his return to the business world.

As I lie in bed watching him, I remember the last time I saw him get ready for work. It was March 2, three and a half weeks before Clare's due date, a morning that felt like any other morning except for one small and seemingly insignificant detail—the dog. Curled up next to me, Spike didn't move when Jeff called her for their morning walk. No matter how enticing and high-pitched he made his *C'mon, girl!* and *Let's go, Spikey!* she remained on the bed, looking nervously at me, her gaze seeking permission to stay put. Giving up on the walk, Jeff approached to kiss me goodbye, and immediately Spike skirted around me and sat facing him, defiant—shielding herself with my large pregnant body. "Weird dog," he said. "She always did love you more." Except for one short trip to the patio to pee, Spike was like a forty-five-pound tumor on my leg that day, moving in tandem with me everywhere I went. When I got up to use the bathroom, she followed. When I got back in bed, she followed. It went on like this right up until Jeff unexpectedly came home in the middle of the afternoon and found me, the dog at my side, resting in the guest bedroom.

"Spike knew," I say to Jeff, who is now sitting on the bed and slipping his feet into black loafers.

"Huh?"

"She tried to warn me with her looks, her clinginess on the day Clare was born. She knew something was up."

Jeff pauses, as if weighing my theory. "Jeez," he says, "you may be right. She was acting pretty strange that morning." He leans back on the bed and ruffles the top of Spike's head, scratches under her chin. "Good girl," he coos, as she revels in his attention. "You're such a good girl."

"Maybe next time she could be more specific."

Setting the phone by my side, Jeff promises to come home for lunch, then kisses me and leaves for work. By the end of the day, he has Matt's blessing to relocate. The next day, I call Mom and ask if she knows a good realtor in Boulder. She does, so I call the realtor and leave a message. The day after, Mom phones to say that she saw a For Sale sign go up in her neighborhood. The house backs up to open space, where deer and foxes regularly roam, and it has a direct view of the foothills that border the Rockies. The location is perfect and the homes on that street rarely go on the market, she tells us, so she'll ask the realtor to check into it.

Jeff and I are percolating with excitement, not just because of the possibility of moving to Mom's neighborhood, but because tonight Clare is coming home. For good. She and Dede are scheduled to land around eight. The plan is for our new nanny, Vi, to join us for dinner and stay with me while Jeff drives to the airport to pick up Dede and Clare. Tomorrow, Dede will teach Jeff and Vi all about Clare's routine, schedule, and idiosyncrasies. My sister-in-law will stay with us through the weekend, ensuring that both Jeff and Vi are comfortable in caring for my daughter. Then Dede will leave, our baby will stay, and at last, we will be a family.

Vi arrives as scheduled and Jeff begins to show her around the house, giving her a crash course on making herself at home. The telephone rings and I overhear Jeff speaking with someone in familiar tones. After hanging up, he comes to the bedroom where I'm resting in the hospital bed, which I still use for naps. "That was Dede," he says. "There are storms in Orange County and her flight is delayed. She'll call back when she knows more."

We have waited this long; a few more hours, perhaps even a day, shouldn't be a problem. But now that the finish line is in sight, now that we have an actual date and time set for Clare's homecoming, this delay feels like an egregious injustice. At nine, Jeff sends Vi home. At ten, I begin crying from exhaustion and Jeff agrees that I should go to bed. I'm too tired to contemplate or even recognize my disappointment over possibly missing Clare's arrival. After helping me settle into bed, Jeff returns to the living room to wait for another update from Dede. I drift off in no time, and my sleep is hard.

Ten hours later I'm jarred awake by the sound of a baby crying. I lie in bed with the same duality of emotion I used to feel as a child on Christmas mornings—wanting to jump from bed to see the gifts under the tree, yet being so tired that falling back to sleep was a likely scenario. Early in my pregnancy, my biggest fear about having a baby was the lack of sleep I'd heard my mom-friends speak of. The thought of waking every few hours to breastfeed or change a diaper frightened me the same way thoughts of the actual birthing process frightened others. Sleep, or the lack thereof, was what made me nervous about sharing my life with an infant. Now, I know there are much worse fears to be had with pregnancy. There is preeclampsia. There is death. And since neither of these was able to stop me, neither will fatigue. I call to Jeff for help getting out of bed. I want to see my baby.

I sit in my lift chair wrapped in blankets, an extra pillow covering my abdomen, which is still sensitive and not fully healed. And resting on that pillow, nestled in the crook of my arm is baby Clare. She's still so tiny, but she's lost that wrinkled Winston Churchill look all newborns seem to share, the look I remember from photographs of her. As she sucks down the bottle of soy formula Dede prepared, she flaps her doughy arms and fisted hands to express her satisfaction. My own arm begins to tire from holding the bottle in place, so Jeff props it up with a stack of throw pillows. *So this is what it's like to feed a baby.* I can do this. I can.

Jeff is in the middle of sharing our Boulder plans with Dede when the phone rings. He answers in the kitchen, and soon I see him pulling out drawers in search of a pencil and paper. He takes notes, allowing the caller to do most of the talking. Between *uh-huh*s, he smiles, exuberant. He hangs up the phone and walks back to the couch but remains standing, too excited to sit.

"You're not going to believe this," he says.

"Try me," I say.

"That house your mom saw for sale? It's officially going on the market this Sunday. They're having an open house at noon that day and the realtor's pretty sure it'll go fast. But she said she could get me in to preview it tomorrow if we want." He pauses, waiting to take in my reaction.

"Tomorrow? How is that even possible?" I say.

"I know. It's crazy, isn't it?" He waits, still hopeful.

"I just don't see how we could do it," I say. "*Tomorrow?*"

"I could fly out early in the morning and be back by bedtime. I could take the video camera and get lots of footage so you could see it, too." He turns toward my sister-in-law. "Dede, if you could watch Clare *and* Lauren ...". Again he waits. My mind is reeling. Neither of us has ever bought a house before. Things are moving too fast.

"I know it's a long shot," he says. "But what if it's perfect for us? What if this is *our* home?"

"I don't mind," Dede says. "We still have the rest of today and all day Sunday to practice Clare's routine together."

I remain speechless, my brain trying to remember how to work fast, juggle logistical details. They both look at me, awaiting my response. Jeff's face implores me to dig deep and find that spontaneity that we both so admired in one another before everything changed.

"I suppose it wouldn't hurt to check on airfares," I say.

I hand the baby to Dede for a diaper change and ask Jeff to bring me the phone. I've always been the planner, the one who has the airline telephone numbers and our frequent-flier numbers memorized. Jeff sits on the couch watching me as I dial United Airlines. A minute later, I hang up the phone without having made a reservation.

"Sixteen hundred," I say. "That's an awful lot of money for a long shot."

Jeff agrees. We sit in silence, and I realize I'm sad about the apparent end to this opportunity.

Then an idea hits me and I dial another number, this one to an automated customer service line. *Maybe, just maybe.* I punch in my eleven-digit frequent-flier number. I didn't do much travel in my last job, but you never know. Next, I punch in my ZIP code.

"Yes!" I say, hanging up the phone and dialing another number, again by heart.

"I have just enough miles for one coach ticket. Now we have to see if they've got availability," I say. The odds that there will be an award-travel seat available are slim. I speak with the customer service representative, telling her the exact flights we need to make this work. When I tell her it's for tomorrow, there's an audible gasp from her end of the line. Then she starts laughing. "Well, what do you know," she says. A minute later, I hang up the phone.

"It's a sign. They had one seat left. You're on the flight." Jeff jumps up from the couch, his excitement unmistakable. Though not as effusive, I'm as thrilled as he is.

The next evening, as Clare sleeps and Dede and I talk in the living room, we hear the sound of a car door slamming, followed by the banging of the security gate on the front porch. Jeff walks through the door, a thick portfolio of paperwork under one arm, his backpack hanging off the other.

"The house is awesome!" he says, leaning over to kiss me. His breath smells of alcohol, no doubt from Mom and John's favorite restaurant.

"You go to The Rio?" I ask.

"Yeah," he says, laughing. "We had to have a margarita before your folks took me back to the airport." Jeff's enthusiasm is obvious as he pulls the camcorder from his backpack and wires it to the television. The day has been a whirlwind of activity for him, a mission really. It makes me feel good to see him so engaged, excited about building our post–train-wreck future. Once the video is ready, he helps me move to the couch so I can see the television. Dede sits on one side, Jeff on the other. He pushes the play button and narrates as the camera moves from room to room in a jerky *Blair Witch* fashion. At times, I must look away because the swift camera movements cause vertigo.

"Look," Jeff says, "here's my office."

"And there's that walk-in closet you've always wanted."

"And look, this is Clare's room."

We finish watching the video and Jeff turns to me. "What do you think?" he asks.

What do I think?

I think my illness has ripped through our lives like an earthquake, decimating the very foundation of all we took for granted, like health and security and faith in our well-orchestrated plans. I think every building block that made up the years of our life together has crumbled into a big heap and we are now free to rebuild it however we damn well please. I think a move to Boulder is exciting and terrifying, and could be good for us and could be bad for us. But mostly, I think it makes me happy to see Jeff so fired up about buying this house, about giving his family a home.

"Let's sign the papers," I say.

For the next thirty minutes, Jeff hands me page after page, pointing to yellow highlighted areas requiring my signature or initials. My grip on the pen is weak, my writing nearly illegible, but I cosign away the bulk of money in our bank account, knowing that this stack of paper represents a new beginning for us. When the last page has been signed, Jeff helps me get to bed before the eight o'clock tears begin. Then he retrieves the fax machine from the garage, sets it up in the dining area, and page by page, transmits our future to a real estate office in Boulder. By the time I wake up the following morning, the sellers have accepted our offer and the Open House sign is removed from the lawn of our new home.

Big changes lie ahead, this time chosen by us.

28

WITH VI'S HELP, WE'VE ESTABLISHED A ROUTINE that is unconventional, yet practical for our extraordinary circumstances. The nanny has temporarily moved in with us so Jeff can sleep through the night rather than awaken every few hours with the baby. Vi sleeps in the twin bed next to Clare's bassinet. And next to Clare is the crib, too big for my baby but perfect for Vi's aging giant rabbit, whose escape is hindered by a window screen acting as a makeshift roof. Jeff leaves for work after giving Clare her first bottle of the day while Vi showers. I sleep until around eleven, then feed Clare while Vi makes me something to eat. Afterward, Vi and Clare head off for their daily date at Starbucks with other nannies and their charges. I picture this small group of twenty-something women exchanging details about their respective clients. "Mine's a Silicon Valley CEO," one might say, stirring her mocha with pride. "Mine's filthy rich, but she's too damn busy with her social engagements and fund-raisers to care for her own kid," another might say, her words dripping with judgment. I imagine Vi holding back, waiting to trump them all with her latest assignment. "Mine came back from the dead."

Vi stands at the door to my bedroom, my baby girl in her arms, a bottle in hand. It's four o'clock and I just woke up from my afternoon nap.

"Clare Bear's ready for her bottle. Would you like to feed her?" Vi asks.

"I'd love to," I say.

I fiddle with the buttons on the hospital bed and make a nest of soft pillows across my belly for Clare. Vi hands me the bottle and settles Clare into my arms. She pulls another pillow from the main bed and tucks it under my bottle-holding arm, giving me enough support to make it through the five minutes it takes Clare to suck down her soy formula. When the bottle is empty, I set it aside and enjoy an unobstructed view of my baby's face. She has this little thing she does immediately after every meal. Her lips continue to move about as if her source of food is still within reach. Then her eyes, wide and alert while there was formula sliding down her throat, begin to get a distant look, her eyelids drooping to half-mast. I speak softly to her, trying out the different monikers bestowed by her Aunt Dede and Uncle Tim and adopted by Vi.

"Hey, Little Monkey. Hi, Clare Bear."

I can hear the uncertainty in my voice, how its inflection is less confident than the nanny's when I eavesdrop on their one-way conversations. I speak in a whisper, perhaps to mask my status as a novice mother, or perhaps to mask the shame that has begun to seep into my thoughts during my waking hours. *Why did all this happen? How is it that I've created such a screwed-up situation for this amazing little being?*

Vi returns and hands me a small plate of my usual—hummus, pita, and raw almonds—then sits on the edge of the other bed to await my next want. Vi is a godsend: capable, caring, and energetic. At twenty-one, she exhibits an ease with newborns that's ten times what mine is at thirty-eight. And she's fabulous with Clare. For that reason alone I feel both gratitude and resentment. Watching her give my baby a bath, listening to her comfort Clare during one of her regular dinnertime crying spells, seeing how efficiently she changes diapers—these all serve to remind me what a failure I am. I'm a mother who can't even mother.

Clare disrupts my despondency with one of her best tricks. While pursing her mouth, her eyes get wide and watery and her face reddens as she holds her breath, no doubt to build the momentum. Then I feel the vibrations through the pillow, hear the rumbling within her tiny purple-flowered pants, and smell the remains of a previous feeding as they exit her bottom.

"Thar she blows!" I say, and Vi and I erupt in appreciative laughter over Clare's scatological comedy routine. Vi lifts Clare from the bed to change her, a look of feigned disgust on her face as she carries my baby from the room at arm's length. For now, my daughter has successfully helped me deflect another bout of self-recrimination.

At dinnertime, Jeff returns from work and changes from his suit to sweatpants and a T-shirt. He and Vi discuss dinner plans as Jeff paces the full length of our tiny home, holding Clare against his chest in an effort to calm her. Like me, she has her own nightly crying period. It begins around six every evening and lasts for several hours. Colic, some of our friends tell us. But I have a different theory, a simple one. She's pissed. For eight months she heard our voices daily, including the bark of her canine sister. Then, nothing. No familiar voices, not one. And just as she adapted to a different maternal presence, it all changed again and the old voices were back. I'd be pissed too.

Jeff sends Vi to pick up sesame chicken, broccoli in garlic sauce, and walnut prawns from Eric's Restaurant on Church Street. When she returns, Jeff and I eat in the living room while Vi bounces the baby on her hip in one of the bedrooms. At just under a thousand square feet, this house is too small to escape the noise of Clare's incessant wailing. Ten minutes into a clamorous meal, Jeff and Vi switch places and roles.

Around eight, Clare's crying begins to wane, brief pauses between piercing fits of anguish. Slowly, the intervals of serenity increase in length until at last—*sweet Jesus*—she is consistently calm. Jeff feeds her a final bottle and then, as Vi puts Clare to bed, Jeff does the same for me. As Vi rocks Clare's bassinet to lull her to sleep, Jeff lulls me with the richness of his voice, reading aloud from a collection of short stories.

Not long into the second chapter, I feel a dull ache begin at the back of my head. Jeff sets the book aside and brings me two Tylenol and some water. I ask him to keep reading to take my mind off the pain, but the magnitude of the throbbing only increases. Soon I'm groaning, then crying. Jeff soaks a washcloth in cold water and holds it against the back of my head. I ask him to turn the lights off, to gently massage my head, to squeeze between my thumbs and forefingers, where the acupressure points that are supposed to eliminate headaches are located. Nothing helps, and the pain intensifies.

I've always been an infrequent headache sufferer and never had a migraine, so this one worries me. I've heard stories of people who've complained of a sudden migraine only to die moments later of a ruptured brain aneurysm. I'm now convinced that's what's happening and it infuriates me—the injustice of surviving all the traumatic events of these past several months only to lose everything in the end, this way. I dare not mention my fears to Jeff. He's been through enough already. Besides, I reason, if it's going to happen, there's no stopping it now.

Jeff asks if he should call an ambulance, but I tell him no, that it's just a really bad headache and there's nothing they can do to help. He continues to cradle my head in the darkness, and the last thought I remember having is *If this is it, please let me go quickly and in my sleep.*

I'm genuinely surprised when I wake up the next morning, my headache replaced by the feeling of being hung over. Jeff hears me stirring and comes to the side of the bed to sit down.

"How're you feeling?" he asks.

"Okay now. That was one hell of a headache."

"You had me worried."

"I didn't want to tell you this last night, but I was certain it was a brain aneurysm or some sort of cerebral blood clot from the seizure I had in the hospital."

"Well, I didn't want to worry *you*, but I went to bed thinking pretty much the same thing."

"I honestly didn't think I was going to wake up today."

We are quiet, each sitting with our private thoughts. Mine focus on how cocky I used to be regarding my health: no broken bones, no hospitalizations, no major illnesses. The compendium of my infirmities over the years includes four ankle sprains, one low-energy semester in college, and an average of one cold per year. Up until two months ago, I simply assumed I would live with vitality well into my nineties, at the very least my late eighties. I've never been a hypochondriac. I was more likely to downplay any medical ailments or symptoms. Where my physical well-being was concerned, I was a lifelong optimist. But now I have a different outlook, one based on fear and mistrust of my body.

29

JEFF HAS A FIRM TWO-HANDED GRIP on my upper right arm while I grasp the railing with my left hand. One step at a time, we make our way down the fifteen stairs between our front door and the sidewalk. Halfway down, we pause so I can catch my breath and regain my balance. We hear Vi behind us and turn to see her standing in the doorway, Clare on her hip.

"Bye, Mom! Bye, Dad!" Vi says, waving our daughter's little hand back and forth.

Jeff and I are going on a date, my first outing since coming home three weeks ago. Until now, I've restricted my visitors to a few close friends, using Jeff as my buffer to the outside world of neighbors, work colleagues, and other friends not in our inner circle. But I'm ready to reengage in the world, starting with an early dinner on 24th Street with another couple, friends of mine from graduate school.

Someone calls to us from across the street, and I look up to see our neighbor jogging toward us, a big smile on his face. Though in his forties and normally low key, Doug looks like a kid who just spotted his parents in the crowd on the last day of summer camp. He clears the steps two at a time until he reaches us, then gives me a light hug.

"Boy, am I glad to see you!" he says.

I feel the same way; am thrilled in fact to reconnect with people who represent my old life. But right now all my energy is focused on merely staying upright, so I let Jeff do the talking while I stand on display—hunched, smiling, and short of breath.

Our neighborhood is composed of a small tight-knit group of families who've lived here since before their children were born. When Jeff and I moved in three years ago, we were the lone renters, the nice professional couple with no children, save for the big black poodle that watched the world from the corner window. Our relationship with the neighbors was limited to cordial greetings, the purchase of candy bars or gift wrap during their children's various school fund-raising events, and for the past two years, an invitation to the annual Robert Burns Dinner hosted by Doug and Christine in honor of Christine's Scottish heritage.

By the time I make it to the bottom of the stairs, two more neighbors, Jody and Claire, have spotted me and are headed in our direction. Jeff snaps a photo of us as we exchange our hellos like long-lost friends. I feel there's been a shift in our relationship, a bond forged from having shared and overcome a difficult challenge. While the illness was all mine, the sense of ownership over supporting my visiting family members was theirs. Just as the neighbors pulled Jeff and me into the communion of their Robert Burns celebrations, we've now pulled them into the communion of our family.

Jeff helps me into the passenger seat of the SUV and drives half a mile to the restaurant as if he's transporting dozens of loose eggs. Our dinner companions have already arrived, and I can see the surprise on their faces when they first set eyes on me. No doubt they've heard how serious my situation was from our mutual friend Pam, but their expressions tell me they expected someone who appeared a bit more, well, normal. They quickly recover their composure and we all follow the hostess to a table in the corner. We are the first diners in the restaurant, having purposely timed it so I can be back home well before my habitual nighttime tears begin. Jeff places the pillow he brought from home on an already padded chair, then lowers me onto the soft seat as if I'm his grandmother instead of his wife. Again, I notice that slight shift in my friends' demeanor, a look, perhaps, of uncertainty about what's appropriate behavior around someone who went toe-to-toe with the grim reaper and survived, though not unscathed. The Lauren they remember was a boisterous, wisecracking fireball who once challenged— and defeated—several grad school classmates in Pac-Man, using her toes to control the joystick while standing on one leg atop a bar stool, beer in one hand, someone's head for balance in the other. This Lauren can barely keep her balance on both feet and looks as if one game of *anything* might put her in the grave.

I order a plate of pasta with cream sauce and a side of sautéed spinach, but partway through my entrée I realize I can no longer sit comfortably. Even with extra cushioning, the bones in my butt are so sore I don't think I can last two more minutes in this chair. Jeff calls for our waiter and asks for the rest of our two meals to be wrapped. We apologize profusely to my friends for having to depart so abruptly, and Jeff pulls his wallet from his pocket.

"No, no," says one of my friends. "This is on us." They both stand and hug us goodbye, and we leave less than an hour after having arrived. I shuffle to the car, Jeff holding onto my arm the whole way, and I can tell I've pushed my body too much. But still, a date.

The following morning, I stay in bed, resting and reading a book about baby care for new parents. Vi has the day off, so Jeff changes Clare's diaper, warms her bottle, and brings both the baby and the bottle to me so I can feed her. He climbs back in bed next to me, and Spike hops up next to him. We are a family of four now, all safely snuggled together on our queen-sized bed. It's a wonderful feeling, and soon Jeff gets up to fetch the camera. He's always been a man who can't simply experience a joyful moment; he must also chronicle it through photos or home video. I've often kidded him about this habit, sometimes been annoyed with the interruption of the camera. Yet when

I peruse the photos or home videos months later, I'm always grateful that he took the time to preserve our life together, our memories. Jeff leans in toward Clare and me, pats the bed for Spike to move in closer, and holds the camera at arm's length, aiming the lens toward the four of us.

"Fromage!" Jeff says, in deference to our mutual love of the south of France.

Years from now when we look at this photo, I'll make fun of the scrawniness of my upper arms and the ropiness of my neck, both lacking any of their former meatiness. Jeff will chide himself for being out of shape from weeks at hospitals instead of the gym. And Clare will adore her own wide-eyed baby face and tiny perfect fingers. Either Jeff or I will mention how interesting it was that Spike's chin turned white during the two months that I was away, and then we'll all say how much we miss her and what a good dog she was. But overriding our commentary about this photograph will be the message it conveys: *We are a family.*

After draining her bottle, Clare falls asleep on the bed. I reach for my journal and flip through it, passing Jeff's notes to get to a blank page. I've written only one other time since coming home, so I'd forgotten about the discovery of my husband's handwriting the same day I found the dried bouquet of roses under the guest bed.

"Why'd you use my journal to take notes at the hospital?" I ask him.

"It was the only paper I had," he says.

"But why did you have my journal *with* you?"

"Because I needed to hear your voice," he says. "I needed to reconnect with you when you were comatose, so I took your journal to the hospital and read it as I sat by your side."

I'm speechless. How awful that must've been for him. How utterly sad and lonely and frightening and heartbreaking.

"It really freaked me out when I read that comment about you waiting for the other shoe to drop," he adds, referencing my fears over the holidays of something bad happening now that my life felt so perfect.

"Wow," I say.

"Yeah, wow."

"Sorry about that," I say, trying to lighten the mood and pull away from the weighty emotions we've inadvertently tapped. "My bad."

"Just don't let it happen again, okay?" His mock anguish is a weak disguise for the pain below the surface.

At lunchtime, Jeff sets his book aside and gets out of bed, where we've spent the entire morning reading, napping, and simply being.

"How 'bout I make us some tostadas," he says.

"Sounds great."

Jeff leaves the room and I hear him bustling about the kitchen, scraping refried beans from a can into a cooking pan, chopping tomatoes and lettuce and onions, opening and closing the squeaky toaster-oven door to heat the tostada shells. Clare is sound asleep by my side on the purple angel quilt that Liz's mom made for her. Spike lies on her back with her hind legs spread-eagled and one of her front legs stretched out straight, a position we call *Charge!* Seeing Spike so at ease, watching my baby girl's mouth move with the little rapid breaths of slumber, and hearing the sounds of mundane life in the kitchen gives me a sense of contentment and peace I haven't felt in a long time. I relish this feeling, this moment.

And suddenly, all hell breaks loose.

The smoke detector's alarm blasts through the house and the odor of something burning permeates the air. Clare is jolted awake and blasts her own alarm of displeasure. Spike leaps off the bed, barking wildly as she sprints toward the kitchen.

"Jeff!" I yell over all the commotion. "What's happening?"
I pull Clare into my arms but am unable to calm her, so she continues to wail at full throttle. Jeff jogs down the hallway, a kitchen towel tossed over his shoulder, spatula in hand. The smoke detector is still blaring in the kitchen.

"The tostada shells are on fire," he says. "Be right back!" He abruptly turns and jogs back down the hallway.

"How serious is it?" I yell. "Do I need to get up? Because I don't think I can while holding Clare!"

The alarm stops blasting and Jeff returns. "I yanked the batteries from the smoke detector," he says. "Here, I can take her."

He lifts Clare, still crying, from my arms and holds her against his chest as he jogs back to the kitchen. I hear him swatting something with a towel and I imagine the scene in the other room: Jeff battling flames with one arm, bouncing a baby with the other. I can't help but laugh. He runs back into the bedroom and hands Clare to me.

"I think I need the fire extinguisher," he says. "Remind me where it is?"

"Under the kitchen sink, to the left," I say. I'm no longer laughing and Clare is still crying. Jeff leaves the room, and soon I hear the discharge of the extinguisher in repeated brief intervals, followed by Jeff coughing, then laughing. I look down the hallway, visible from my side of the bed, and see my husband walking toward me, fire extinguisher in hand, residual smoke clinging to the ceiling overhead.

"Well," he says, holding up the fire extinguisher, "at least we know it works!" He drops the heavy red cylinder in the corner and picks up Clare again, bouncing her as he walks back and forth across the bedroom. At last her crying subsides, and Jeff sits on the edge of the bed next to me.

"How about pizza delivery?" he asks, and we both laugh.

30

"Here, honey," Jeff says to me. "It's your very first Mother's Day card."

Tears slide down my cheeks, a mixture of joy and sorrow. I am a mother. And yet, not fully.

"I wish I had more of a celebration lined up," Jeff says. "Since Vi's spending the day with her family, I didn't make any big plans." The idea of Jeff trying to manage an outing with both Clare and me seems laughable. Quiet time at home with no kitchen fires, minimal crying from Clare, and maybe a movie rental will be celebration enough for me. The phone rings and Jeff runs to the kitchen to answer it. He returns minutes later, a big smile on his face.

"Katherine just offered to babysit Clare," he says. "I can take you to a Mother's Day brunch after all."

I've been out for only two restaurant meals since coming home: the dinner with my grad school friends and another dinner after a follow-up appointment with Keyser Söze, during which he told Jeff and me we could "resume relations." (We both choked back guffaws; the thought of even trying to have sex again seemed absurd.) Physical discomfort aborted both meals long before our waiters could tempt us with a dessert menu, so I'm not really interested in testing the third-time's-a-charm theory. But Jeff seems determined to make this day a special one and I don't want to dampen his enthusiasm.

"Sounds great," I say.

I get out of bed, do my bathroom routine, and get dressed—all without help. We hear Clare fussing, and since I'm still unable to lift her from her bassinet or carry her, I settle into the lift chair while Jeff retrieves her. He places her on my lap and then brings a warm bottle. As I feed Clare, Jeff calls various restaurants in hopes of securing a coveted reservation for brunch. One Market, Campton Place, and Top of the Mark are all booked, he tells me after a few phone calls.

"I even tried using the 'my wife almost died in childbirth' line," he says. "Didn't work."

"Tough crowd," I say. Secretly, I'm relieved that I may not have to sit still, and in likely discomfort, for several hours at a restaurant. There's a knock at the door and Katherine lets herself in. She comes to my lift chair and coos over Clare before turning her attention to Jeff.

"So where are you taking her?" she asks.

"Right now, nowhere. I can't find one damn restaurant with an opening," Jeff says. He turns to me. "I'm sorry, hon. I'm striking out here." He looks truly crestfallen, like he's failed me.

"That's okay," I say. "You know where I *really* feel like going?"

"Where?"

"Costco."

The look on both of their faces is priceless.

"You're kidding, right?" asks Jeff.

"I'm not. I want to do something normal, like shop for toilet paper and dog treats."

"Really?"

"Really. Besides, this is probably the one time I can drag you there and you won't complain."

"Well, you got that right. Costco it is."

An hour later, wearing a pair of my husband's sweatpants and a ratty old sweatshirt, I shuffle up and down warehouse aisles, steadying myself with one hand on the side of the oversized shopping cart Jeff is pushing. I point to cases of bottled water and jumbo boxes of Goldfish crackers and two-packs of extra-virgin olive oil, and without a hint of annoyance, Jeff loads each item into our cart. After checking out, we order hot dogs and sodas at the Costco cafeteria. Sitting at one of the indoor picnic tables, we eat our Mother's Day "brunch," saving part of each hot dog for Spike, who's waiting in the car. Right now, I couldn't be any happier. I feel ordinary. And ordinary, I'm learning, can be wonderful.

Two weeks later, it's Jeff's fortieth birthday and my turn to host a special outing. My apprehension about dining out has dissipated, so Liz and Sabra have helped me make arrangements for a surprise party at Vivace Ristorante, an old favorite haunt from my days in suburbia. I ate there once and sometimes twice a week when I lived close by, and even after moving to the city, Jeff and I made the half-hour trek south on a regular basis. Early in my pregnancy, the restaurant's owner, Michael, told me that he and his wife were expecting their first child too, so we often spoke of how excited we both were to become parents. And later, while I was in the hospital, Sabra stopped by to pick up an order of my favorite dish—gnocchi in Gorgonzola cream sauce—hoping it would encourage me to eat. Michael refused payment, sending his best wishes with the to-go bag.

To quell any suspicions, I've told Jeff that Liz, Rick, and I are taking him out to dinner for his birthday. At six, we arrive at Vivace and Michael greets us at the door. Again I notice that subtle shift in facial features whenever someone I know sees me for the first time since my illness. It's an expression that either says *I'm sorry for what you've been through* or *Holy cow, you look awful!* Maybe both. My weight is back to normal—150 pounds—but my skin remains bronze, my posture stooped. Michael quickly recovers his composure and gives me a familial kiss on the cheek.

"It's been a long time," he says.

"Over three months," I say. "I'm guessing that's an all-time record for me."

Michael shakes hands with Liz and Rick, whom he recognizes as friends of ours from other Vivace visits, and then he shakes Jeff's hand, holding on a bit longer than is customary.

"Table for four?" Michael asks.

"Yes, thanks," Jeff says. And that's when I know we've truly fooled him.

"I have the perfect one," Michael says. He leads us toward the heavy velvet drapes that separate the restaurant's main dining area from the more intimate back room. Pulling back the curtain, he reveals helium balloons and streamers, a pile of brightly wrapped gifts, and a dozen of our friends wearing party hats and giddy grins.

"Surprise!" they yell, tossing confetti and twirling noisemakers, which add a cacophonous stone-on-cheese-grater sound to the clamor. Jeff looks flummoxed. We join our friends and all take seats at one huge table. Sabra places an enormous red-and-gold crown on Jeff's head while Liz, Rick, and I put on our less extravagant party hats like those the rest of the guests are already wearing. Waiters pour champagne—soda for me—and toasts are made, many reflecting the recent hardships that Jeff has conquered to make it to this birthday. Raucous jokes and sincere sentiments mix easily throughout the conversation as we share a family-style meal of calamari, smoked salmon, Caesar salad, linguini with clams, lamb shank, sautéed spinach, and of course, gnocchi in Gorgonzola cream sauce.

Waiters replace the dirty dinner plates with generous portions of creamy tiramisu and we all sing "Happy Birthday" off-key. I bask in the camaraderie of this "chosen family" Jeff and I have developed, a potpourri of friends collected during different phases of our life. I luxuriate in Sabra's balls-out laugh at something Liz just whispered in her ear. Margaret's mannerisms suggest she drank too much, while Dean's, not enough.

Peter is coaxing Jeff to go on one last backpacking trip before we move to Colorado, the two of them recounting past nature retreats with bravado, an excess of wine turning peaks they've climbed into twice their actual elevation. From the far end of the table, Ilene lets loose her Muppet-like laugh, and Jennine's voice carries across the room, while her husband, Chris, holds back, content to let her have center stage. The people at this table are no longer *Jeff's* friends or *Lauren's* friends, but are *our* friends. Over the years, we've shared food and wine, jazz concerts and movies, camping trips and spa trips. Now, we have another shared experience to add to our repertoire—near-fatal preeclampsia. I know beyond a doubt that the people honoring my husband tonight are with us through thick and thin, and that none of the still-wrapped gifts they've brought could possibly trump the gift of their friendship.

Over the next several weeks, life takes on a sense of normalcy. My physical recovery still has a long way to go, but the focus at home has shifted from health challenges to parenting challenges—namely, how to calm a baby who cries nonstop from sundown till bedtime.

It's nearing dinnertime on a Sunday and we're driving to the In-N-Out Burger in Petaluma. Thirty-eight miles seems a bit far to go for a drive-through burger, especially when there's another In-N-Out in the city less than five miles from our home. But it's not our favorite burgers and shakes that Jeff and I crave. It's peace, a respite from Clare's wailing, which seems to have been going on for hours by the time Jeff straps her car seat into the back of the SUV. Riding in the car, someone told us, is one of the best ways to calm a crying baby. By the time we hit the Golden Gate Bridge, Clare is asleep. Even Spike, sitting unobtrusively next to her new sister, seems to understand that we should all be careful not to speak or we'll wake the baby and suffer the consequences.

I use this quiet time to admire the calendar-photo views of the city I've called home twice: the Marina, Alcatraz Island, the flicker of sunlight off the bay. In 1986, I left San Francisco the first time for graduate school in Los Angeles. Before driving out of town in my secondhand '68 VW Squareback, I wrote a list of goals I wanted to accomplish in the next ten years. Among them was to be living in San Francisco again.

One month shy of my deadline I moved back to San Francisco, having accomplished every goal on my list but one: being happily married. At the time, I was quite at ease with my potential status as a lifelong single woman. I had plenty of friends, a busy social life, and a faithful, albeit irreverent, canine companion. I had no idea that months after settling in the Bay Area for the second time, my Prince Charming would—quite literally—show up at my doorstep, and that two business meetings and two dates later, we'd be engaged. But our story didn't end with the classic fairytale happily-ever-after. We were tested beyond anything we could've imagined, and now the battle is over. Though individually wearied, as a couple we've been strengthened in ways we have yet to fully comprehend.

I gaze at San Francisco Bay, the sun now setting over the Pacific. This landscape has always caused me to catch my breath, made me believe I'm one of the luckiest people on earth by virtue of living here. Yet in one month, we'll leave this place for a new beginning in the Rocky Mountains. I'm exhilarated by the excitement change offers, yet simultaneously reluctant to abandon the place that has felt like the first real home I've had since leaving Wenonah, the one-square-mile town in South Jersey where I was born and raised.

As Clare continues sleeping, we pass through Sausalito, where Jeff and I stopped for lunch during an all-day bike ride shortly after moving from the suburbs to the city. We drive through the Waldo Tunnel with its faded mural of a rainbow running along the arch at the entrance. Normally, we'd toot the horn halfway through the tunnel, signaling Spike to offer a bark or two. Instead, I turn to Jeff and mouth *beep-beep* while mimicking leaning on a car horn, and Spike remains quiet.

We pass the exit for Tiburon, where we'd spent several Sunday afternoons on the outdoor patio of a bayside Mexican restaurant, sipping margaritas in the sunshine before taking the ferry back to the city.

Six more miles down the highway, the sign for Larkspur transports me back to our first New Year's Eve together. Jeff had told me to show up at a particular address in the city at six o'clock sharp wearing something flapper-style. He gave me no other details about our evening other than to say, "Trust me." When I arrived via cab in my fringed and feathered getup, a red boa around my neck, he stepped out of a martini bar to greet me, zoot suit and all. After one cocktail in a crowded lounge of normally dressed people, he took me to an upscale restaurant in Larkspur that had transformed itself into a speakeasy for the evening. We gave the secret password at the door, entered, and were served a five-course meal that was interrupted with a staged gangster-style shoot-out. Later, we went to an elegant little inn where Jeff had already registered us, supplying all I would need for an evening away and having made dog-sitting arrangements for Spike. It was after making love the following morning that we talked about our future and decided that someday we'd move to Boulder. He'd fallen in love with the area during his first visit there to meet my mom and stepdad. *Someday, Boulder* became our mantra.

A few more miles down the highway we pass the turnoff for Nicasio, the little town nestled among redwoods where Jeff and I were married. We'd rented the vacation compound of a Hollywood producer, housed our immediate family in the guest cottages, and exchanged vows in a rustic outdoor amphitheater before dancing under the stars to Chris's eighteen-piece jazz orchestra. I'm tempted to suggest that we drive the ten miles out of our way to see if the sapling we planted on the morning of our wedding day is still alive, but since it's the weekend, the owner's family is most likely enjoying their home away from home. We continue the drive in glorious silence.

At last we reach the exit for In-N-Out Burger and Jeff pulls up to the drive-through menu board. We whisper our orders: two Double Doubles with cheese, fries, a vanilla milk shake for Jeff, a Pepsi for me. Remarkably, the restaurant employee's loud and tinny voice fails to awaken our daughter when he repeats our order over the intercom. Jeff advances to the next window, hands me our food while paying for our burgers, and then pulls into a vacant parking space, leaving the car idling. One satisfying bite into our meal, Clare stirs, opens her eyes, and launches into another round of wailing.

"Unfuckingbelievable," Jeff says.

He sets his burger on the dashboard and reaches into the backseat for the baby bottle he packed. We're laughing, but our ability to see the humor in these consistent crying spells is waning. Bottle in hand, Jeff tilts his car seat back and leans in toward Clare. He holds the bottle in place for her and she quickly shifts from crying to sucking. I continue to eat my burger, albeit more quickly, and soon Jeff and I switch roles, with me feeding Clare while he wolfs his food down. We know we must finish our burgers before Clare finishes her bottle or risk eating to a cacophony of bawling. Minutes later, Clare drains the last of the formula and the wailing begins.

"I can't take it," Jeff says. "Let's just go, okay?"

"Fine by me," I say.

We both reach back and feed the last bit of our burgers to Spike before tossing the rest of the fries and our drinks in the trash. We pull back onto the highway for the long ride home, and within minutes Clare is sound asleep. With a good ten miles remaining in our commute, we hear the telltale rumble from our baby's bottom, but neither of us suggests we stop for a diaper change. The silence is too precious to disturb.

31

IT'S BEEN ALMOST TWO MONTHS since my release from the
hospital and I'm about to embark on my first big test. Vi is
out of town for a week and Jeff leaves in less than an hour for
three nights away, his first business trip in months. He's asked
me no less than ten times if I'm sure I can handle this. Yes, I've
said repeatedly, knowing the real answer was no. I'm anything
but sure. My feet, knees, elbows, and hands ache constantly, as
if from severe arthritis, and I run out of physical steam quickly.
But at some point I have to step up to the plate. Nervous, but
determined, I know it's time for me to be my child's mother in
more than name only.

After showering and dressing, Jeff changes Clare's overnight
diaper, makes her a bottle, and hands both the baby and the
bottle to me in the bed. He packs his suitcase while I feed our
daughter. When Clare has finished and pooped, Jeff changes
her diaper again before handing her back to me, kissing me
goodbye, and asking one last time if I'll be all right.

"Go!" I say, putting forth my best *quit worrying* persona. Part
of me believes my own display of aplomb. For most of my life
when my doubts said I couldn't, I squelched them by adopting
an air of overconfidence. Instead of running a half-marathon, I
signed up for the full 26.2 miles, though I'd completed only one
10K at that point in my running career. Instead of accepting
the director-level position, I'd interview for the job, then ne-

gotiate for the vice-presidency. And instead of simply joining a club and settling in as a new member, I'd join and immediately run for president. So far this technique has served me well in overcoming my fears. But marathons, jobs, and extracurricular activities are no match for babies. Still, I cling to my bravado with a certainty that convinces both Jeff and me. Besides, what I lack in physical ability I make up for in friendships. Patt, a former work colleague, has offered to stay with me while my husband is out of town. She has to put in a full day at the office, she told me, but she'll be here by five-thirty tonight.

Jeff leaves for the airport and I get out of bed to dress. My wardrobe remains quite limited: loose-fitting sweatpants, one of Jeff's button-down shirts, and flat, heavily cushioned shoes. Clare and I have an appointment in Berkeley in less than two hours, one I purposely neglected to mention to my husband. I began driving again a week ago, but only to and from the pool where I swim five to ten laps each day. My driving is precarious, my neck too stiff to completely rotate toward the car's blind spots. I either have to trust the side-view mirrors or turn my entire upper body before changing lanes, which often jerks the steering wheel a bit off course. Today is the first time I'll be driving with my baby in the car, a plan I know Jeff would vehemently oppose.

While Clare naps, I pack her diaper bag with supplies for the next four hours: two prepared bottles in a heat-retaining sac, diapers, wipes, a spit cloth, and a spare outfit in case of a "blowout." I put the diaper bag on the table by the door and collect other necessities for the trip: bottled water, my purse, ibuprofen in case my joints begin to ache too much, and the driving directions that were dictated over the phone when I set the appointment a few days ago. Spike hears the jingle of car keys and excitedly jumps off the couch, tail wagging as she heads toward me.

"Sorry, Spikey," I tell her. "Can't take you this time."

Ever since I adopted Spike when she was seven weeks old, she has gone almost everywhere in the car with me: on errands, on road trips for work and pleasure, to the office on weekends. The car is like a doghouse on wheels to Spike, a place where she is both comfortable and comforted. When I was two months pregnant, she went car camping with Jeff and me along the northern California coastline. After the sun had set, she was too nervous to sit outside by the campfire with us, so we put her in the car, the window halfway open, with a direct view of our campsite. She relaxed immediately, so we left her there until we all went to sleep inside the tent hours later.

But today is different. I'm nervous enough about driving with Clare across the heavily trafficked Bay Bridge, about venturing farther than the pool. Spike is seven years old, trained to walk off leash, and predictable in her behavior, but the small risk of her disobeying and running off, or pulling me if I leash her, is beyond my physical capabilities. She looks dejected, her tail drooping as she returns to the couch. *You weren't like this before that furless puppy came to live with us,* her body language seems to say.

I have everything I need for the trip piled on the table. I lift Clare from her bassinet to the changing table and give her a fresh diaper for the ride. She remains sleepy and agreeable as I settle her into the portable car seat and strap her in. Then I stand at the doorway and try to decide how best to load Clare, the diaper bag, and my purse into the car. I have gone up and down the stairs many times by now, but never with anything in my arms, let alone a baby. I realize how dependent I've become on Jeff handling all the little details, even loading my lightweight swim bag for me whenever I head to the pool. Fear rises in my throat as I debate which path to the car would be best—through the garage or through the front door. Which railing is sturdier, I wonder, in case I stumble and must rely on it to keep my baby and me from tumbling down the remaining stairs? Should I load the baby first or the supplies? Carrying Clare in her car seat in one hand and the diaper bag and purse in the other is not an option. I need at least one hand free for the railing. What if I load Clare first and return to the house for the supplies only to realize my energy is depleted and my baby is trapped fifteen steps below in the car? What if I load the supplies first and then don't have the energy to get back up the stairs to Clare? Never during pregnancy did I imagine that a simple car trip with a baby would present such a challenge. I consider calling the whole thing off.

"You can do this, Lauren," I hear myself say aloud.

I decide to load the diaper bag and purse first, getting to the car by way of the indoor staircase. Clare naps quietly in her car seat atop the dining room table as I make my way down to the garage. I load the car, back it out into the short driveway, turn off the ignition, and lock the doors lest I lose my energy once back inside the house. I come back to the living room through the front door and am delighted, if not a bit surprised, to see Clare still safely asleep in the same spot. I rest on the couch and pet Spike for a few minutes before round two. When I feel ready, I push myself up from the couch and take the baby car seat by the handle. I make it out the front door and to the top of the stairs, and then I freeze. *I can't do this, I can't do this, I can't do this* runs through my head.

"You *can* do this, Lauren," I say again.

My legs are shaking with the same precarious feeling that comes with trying to remain standing after crossing the finish line of a marathon, when your body says simply *Done*. I'm torn between not wanting any of the neighbors to see me so frightened and wishing like hell they'd come to my rescue. I stand frozen in place and nearly in tears; then I finally bend my left leg and allow my right foot to reach downward for the step below. The palms of my hands are sweating from the strength of my grip on both the railing and the car seat handle. I make it down one stair and release a huge gust of breath through my mouth. *I can do this, I can do this, I can do this* I say to myself for the next fourteen steps. Once on the sidewalk, I send my version of a silent prayer to unseen forces. *Thank you.*

I load Clare into the backseat of the SUV, start the car, and make my way through San Francisco, across the bridge and toward the address on the sheet of directions. The drive is, by choice, slow and uneventful. When I pull into the driveway of an understated home on a quiet street, Dusa walks out a side door to meet me.

"You made it," she says, wrapping me in a hug. "Can I help you with the baby?" she asks, already poking into the backseat.

I follow her into her colleague's home office, where three other women await. Introductions are made. These women all share the same look of inner peace that Dusa radiates, a gentle aura of being okay with what is versus struggling against what isn't. They wear a variety of clothing and jewelry that screams New Age to me: stones and crystals and gauzy fabrics in loose-fitting designs. None wears makeup or perfume. Their hair is simply styled or not styled at all. They all look, well, uncomplicated—and happier than I ever looked when I was battling my way up every rung of the corporate ladder.

One of the women leads me to a massage table and instructs me to remove my clothes and lie on my back. There's no expectation that I require privacy, no sense that modesty is called for. After all the exposure my body had while in the hospital, I disrobe without a thought and lie on the table. Across the room, Dusa releases the safety buckles across Clare's chest and lifts her from the car seat.

"Are you okay if I remove her clothing, Lauren?" she asks.

"Sure," I say.

Dusa carries my naked little girl, now awake, toward me and gently lays her on my chest, well above my surgical scars. Two of the women lift the sheets hanging down from the table up over Clare and me, careful to leave our heads exposed for ease of breathing. Then all four women encircle the table and begin placing their hands on seemingly predetermined points: my head, arms, and feet, Clare's back. Dusa has already told me that the goal of this treatment is to reconnect the energetic mother-baby bond that was swiftly and abruptly severed at Clare's birth through both the unexpected C-section and the ensuing two-month separation.

It's a little freaky, this four-person hands-on healing session, but as a convert to Dusa's unconventional techniques, I question nothing. I trust her, and her colleagues, implicitly. Clare is quiet for a few minutes and then she starts to cry. The crying quickly morphs to wailing, but none of the women says or does anything to indicate that we need to interrupt the process. Instead, they keep their hands in place on our bodies and encourage Clare to say whatever she has to say.

"That's right," Dusa says. "Get it all out, little one."

"Yes," another woman says. "Of course that made you mad."

My eyes are closed and the soothing voices of these women calm me despite the volume of Clare's howls. I feel neither annoyance nor embarrassment over her outburst, just compassion for all that she's been through. I've spent almost four months focused on the pain this illness caused me. Now, in this moment, every ounce of my being is focused on the pain it caused my baby, a pain I suspect she will never recall on a conscious level, but one that may forever be embedded in her subconscious. I make no move to wipe away my tears as they stream steadily toward my ears. I don't open my eyes when someone blots the sides of my face with a tissue. Instead, I mouth the words *thank you* and realize I'm crying even harder at the simplicity of her kindness. The love I feel in the care of these four women—three of them strangers less than an hour ago—is almost too much to bear. Clare must feel it as well because within minutes her wailing ceases. Usually when a crying spell begins, it lasts until she wears herself out—two, maybe three hours. There is no noise now except the soft and continuous encouragement from the women.

I open my eyes to check on Clare and there she is, eyes open, curiously looking about the room, at peace against my chest. I close my eyes again, no longer crying but grateful. Grateful for experiences such as this, which I would've scoffed at and smugly rejected not so long ago. But illness has taught me humility and openness and acceptance. And right now it feels good to allow these women to heal, reconnect, or strengthen whatever energy may or may not exist on some subtle level of my being that may or may not exist.

The session lasts for two hours, and when it's over I'm simultaneously wiped out and energized, as after waking from a long sleep when the body has not fully engaged in the conscious world. Clare's tranquillity is still intact, and minutes after I buckle her into the car seat, she falls asleep. The drive home is without incident. I pull into the garage and sit in the car an extra minute, lauding myself for successfully managing an outing with my baby all by myself. I detach Clare's car seat from its base and carry it up the stairs to the living room, leaving the diaper bag in the car. The trip has drained me, and right now I want nothing more than to climb into bed and take a nap before Patt arrives at dinnertime.

Spike wags her tail when she sees us but is remarkably subdued and remains on the couch. This response is usually reserved either for when she's sick or has gotten into trouble, as if she thinks that by being less effusive we won't notice the contents of the kitchen trash can strewn about the floor. But the cabinet door to the trash can remains shut and the kitchen is in order. Maybe she's still pissed that I didn't take her with us, I think, making my way down the hallway toward the bedrooms. Spike doesn't follow us. I stop at Clare's room to transfer her from her car seat to the bassinet, and instantly it's clear, the reason for Spike's evasiveness. The two-foot-tall Diaper Genie, with its patented dog-proof lid, has been tipped over and is wide open. Pieces of soiled disposable diapers are strewn about the floor. Complicating the mess are all the tiny absorbency beads from the diaper crotches, saturated with urine and scattered across the carpeting like a sea of aqua-colored caviar. Spike has had quite the party while we were gone.

I put Clare in her bassinet without waking her and bend to pick up the diaper scraps, shoving them back into the Diaper Genie. I quietly curse Spike for making this mess and chide myself for not closing the lid properly in the first place. The Diaper Genie has never been violated during Jeff's or Vi's watch. I walk to my bedroom and stop cold at the doorway. There are more pieces of diaper, more absorbency beads all over the bed, and my velvet duvet is splattered with baby poop.

I can't even handle being on my own for one fucking day!

Crying, I yank the corners of the blanket into the center of the bed, folding it into a giant shit burrito. Still crying, I carry it down the hallway, open the front door, and hurl it onto the brick walkway of our tiny entry area. I have no energy to deal with it today. I return to the bedroom and lie down, covering myself with the small throw blanket that Jeff gave me as a gift the day after I left the hospital. Spike enters the bedroom, tail between her legs, to seek forgiveness and cuddling, and I send her away with a sharp scolding.

After napping for an hour, I awaken, still cranky, when Patt lets herself in using the key I left under the welcome mat for her. She comes down the hallway and stands in the bedroom doorway, suitcase in hand, wearing a tailored business suit and looking like a modern-day Mary Poppins.

"From the looks of the front porch, it appears my first task is to go to the Laundromat!" Patt says, following her pronouncement with a boisterous laugh.

Even though she was far more senior than I when we worked together in publishing, there isn't one hint in her voice or demeanor that it is beneath her to wash my bedcovers. Her competence, as both a mother who raised two kids and an executive who reentered the business world after her divorce, is a godsend. She scoops Clare from her bassinet, changes her diaper, and carries her out the door for the trip to the laundry.

Two hours later, Patt returns with a happy baby, a clean duvet and down blanket, and an aromatic bag of Chinese take-out. I start to get up from the couch, but she signals for me to stay seated. She hands me my baby and begins rummaging through the kitchen for napkins and utensils, returning with a plate of food for me. As I eat, Patt gently swings my baby back and forth, as if Clare is flying across the airspace in front of her, then flying in reverse to begin the game again. I laugh each time Clare smiles as she is thrust forward, and I set my plate aside to get the camera. After snapping a few photos, I realize it's 7:30 and Clare isn't wailing. This is the first night she's been home that she hasn't launched into a lengthy crying spell. When we all go to sleep a couple of hours later, she's still calm.

The following morning, I awaken to find Patt once more standing in my bedroom doorway, wearing a different business suit and bouncing Clare on her hip. "Here you go," she says, handing me a warm bottle of formula and my daughter. "Gotta run." She looks rested, even buoyant.

"You aren't tired? You managed to sleep last night?" I ask, still disbelieving the image of my friend looking so refreshed after sleeping two feet from Clare's bassinet.

"She didn't wake up even once," Patt says. "She slept, well, like a baby!" She laughs at her own joke, turns, and walks from the room.

"See you again tonight," she yells, and I hear the front door click shut.

For the next two days, Patt brings me dinner, rocks my baby at night, and provides much-needed adult conversation at the end of the day. When Jeff returns on Thursday, he finds a clean house and dinner waiting. Scanning this tranquil domestic scene, his face emanates relief, as if he expected to find utter mayhem upon his return. We sit together at the small dining table and share spinach, rice, and lentils while Clare gently vibrates in her battery-operated bouncy seat, a pacifier in her mouth. Halfway through the meal, Jeff sets down his glass of red wine and looks at Clare, then at me.

"What's up with her?" he asks.

"What do you mean?" I say, though I know perfectly well what he means. I want to hear him say it, to confirm that the subtle transformation I've witnessed in our daughter's disposition is neither wishful thinking nor a figment of my imagination.

"She's so … calm!" he says. "It's like something's shifted."

"It has," I say. "And you can thank Dusa."

32

"Damn, my hair is gorgeous," I say.

"It sure is," Mom replies, admiring the auburn tint of my shoulder-length locks, a fortuitous result of liver failure, sort of jaundice for hair.

"I guess this is one silver lining of the train wreck."

"Hell of a way to change your hair color, though."

Mom is back in San Francisco for the weekend to attend Sabra's party. Possessing exquisite taste in all matters related to home and hearth, Sabra decided it was time to do what Southern girls like her do best—host a luncheon. The guest list includes a small group of women who were intimately involved in my ordeal: Katherine and Carrie, both of whom organized blood drives; Nina, whose food brigade kept my family fed; Liz and Pam, who regularly took the eight o'clock and midnight shifts with me while I was in the ICU; and Mom, deserving of an invitation for no other reason than she survived the near death of her youngest child.

It's been more than two months since my discharge, and I'm ready for a little fun with my gal pals. I look pretty darn good, considering. The greasiness of my skin has subsided, leaving me with what looks like a dark tan. The whites of my eyes have lost some of their yellow tint. My weight has dropped considerably, though my scarred belly hangs over my pubic bone, creating a muffin top without the help of tight jeans. Loose-fitting clothing, still a necessity, offers the added benefit of covering the puffiness of my gut and the boniness of my limbs. And I'm still hunched, my shoulders curving inward as if to protect my heart. But what about my hair? It's now shiny, auburn, and straight. In a word, gorgeous.

Jeff, Clare, and Spike are preparing to leave for their walk to the coffee shop on 24th Street as Mom and I pull out of the driveway. Waving goodbye through the car window, I take a minute to savor the scene on the sidewalk. My husband, *The New Yorker* magazine tucked under his arm, his favorite leather baseball cap on his head. My baby, wearing her purple and green flower-print pants and a solid purple onesie, a pacifier— or *binky*, as we call it—in her mouth, fists pumping wildly as Jeff straps her into the stroller with extra-tall handles. And my dog, one of her signature bandanas around her neck, prancing behind Jeff in anticipation, as if to say *Let's go! Let's go! Time for walkies! Let's go!* It looks commonplace, like an everyday father-daughter-dog outing. It looks like love.

Mom pulls up to the curb outside Sabra's home and helps me out of the car before driving away to find parking. I wait for her to return and she helps me up the stairs to the front door.

Once inside, I hug each of my friends, who are all clapping at my arrival. We move to Sabra's dining room and I survey my surroundings: the beautiful serving table filled with silver and cut-glass dishes, the linen table runner and napkins, the china place settings. It's classic Sabra, no less breathtaking in its artistry than the floral arrangements she created for my wedding. Then I notice the place cards adorned with frogs—artistic, tasteful in fact, but *frogs* nonetheless. And under the serving dishes: *lily pads*.

The *pièce de résistance*, the party element that pushes me to the brink of peeing myself with laughter, is the large poster, designed and printed by Sabra's artist husband, also adorned with frogs and lily pads. In large lettering, the caption reads *Thank God Lauren Didn't Croak.*

Sabra waltzes in from the kitchen holding another serving platter. "Did y'all notice the food?" she asks, obviously pleased with her party motif. "D'y'all know how hard it is to plan an entire menu of green cuisine?" We sit down to feast on chilled cucumber soup, salad with avocados and green grapes, and pistachio cake with green cream-cheese frosting, and we make toast after toast with sparkling lime punch. My Rainbow Girl has done it again.

Fingering the back of my head, I wonder why it feels like rubber. *Rubber? On my head?*

It's one, maybe two in the morning, a week after Sabra's luncheon, and I dig through the middle drawer of the bathroom vanity, finally pulling out the hand mirror that once belonged to my grandmother. Holding it to my face, I look at the back of my head in the larger mirror over the sink.

What the hell?

It looks like rubber, flesh-colored rubber about the size of a quarter, right where my head hits the pillow. *A damn bald spot!*

I was so proud of myself for getting out of bed to pee without having to wake Jeff for help. Clearly, I've shifted from survival mode to recovery mode. But going bald? No one warned me about this. I need to talk to Jeff about this rubbery spot on my head, need to confirm that what I see is, in fact, what's there. I make my way back to the bedroom and stand in the dark beside my sleeping husband.

"Hon," I whisper. "Honey, wake up."

"Wha'… ? What!" Jeff says, jerking his body upright, the urgency in his voice a sign that he's still on high alert.

"I'm sorry. I know this sounds stupid, but I think I'm going bald. Can you come look?"

Jeff rubs the sleep from his eyes and follows me back down the dark hallway. Taking a minute to allow his eyes to adjust to the bright lights of the bathroom, he leans in toward the back of my head and moves a bit of my hair out of the way.

"Yep," he says. "That's a bald spot."

He hugs me, then pulls back, placing his hands on my shoulders and looking me in the eyes. I can tell he's assessing my mood, trying to determine if a bit of levity will help or harm. "When we got married, I promised I'd stick with you through thick and thin," he says. "That includes your hair." He laughs at his own joke and I pretend to be annoyed.

"Hey, c'mon," he says. "It's nothing to wig out over." I make a show of groaning, but Jeff is on a roll. "You know what they say—hair today, gone tomorrow!"

He kisses me goodnight and leaves me alone in the bathroom to ponder my impending hairlessness. I pick up the hand mirror to examine the bald spot again. I tug at a small clump of hair and it comes out effortlessly. I turn out the light and hobble back to the bedroom.

The next day I contact several doctors—my obstetrician, liver specialist, hematologist—to ask if they know why I'm losing my hair. They're all stumped, but to be fair, the only other case of preeclampsia they'd seen that was as dramatic as mine had occurred years before. And instead of losing her hair, the patient lost her life.

Going bald seems to be yet another of my body's strategies for ridding itself of built-up toxins, similar to my greasy Wolf Girl stage, or during my last two weeks in the hospital when my skin was dry, almost reptilian, and came off in big sheets, the kind my family used to love tugging at after we'd gotten sunburned during day trips to the Jersey shore. On one occasion, I awoke from a nap in the hospital to find my mother and sister actually having a skin-peeling contest, lurking over me like a couple of vultures picking at their prey.

Early on, I'm able to disguise my hair loss through careful combing and the strategic placement of barrettes and ponytails. Most people I encounter either don't notice my baldness or pretend not to. I swim regularly at the community pool and shower in the locker room after. Accepting that there's no saving my hair, I've begun combing my fingers through it and removing clumps of it while I shampoo each day. Often, I'm alone in the locker room, but today there's someone showering next to me. Adhering to the unspoken mores of gang showers, neither of us strikes up a conversation.

As I shampoo, I carefully pull fistful after fistful of loose hair from my head, setting each clump on a paper towel on the countertop nearby to avoid clogging the shower drain. From the corner of my eye I see the other woman staring at me, clearly aghast. Pretending not to notice, I say nothing to explain myself. I'm rather enjoying this. Several minutes pass and her sideways glances at me continue, so I decide to have a little fun at her expense. Removing another fistful of hair, I hold it out toward her and deadpan, "Does the chlorine level in the pool do this to *your* hair too?"

The look on her face is priceless. And I never see her at the pool again.

It's moving day, July 26, and we're awaiting the arrival of Peseti and his cousin, whom we've hired to help with the relocation to Boulder. Having met Peseti through work years ago, I'm aware of his massive build and corresponding strength. I'm hopeful that these two Tongans, with the aid of my husband, will be able to load our furniture and boxes by day's end. The screeching of truck brakes calls me to the window, and I look out to see a twenty-four-foot U-Haul pull up to the curb. Peseti jumps down from the driver's side, while his wife exits through the passenger door. She's agreed to help clean the house after our things are removed. A pickup truck with four more Tongans pulls up, extra help I hadn't planned on. Peseti throws open the back of the U-Haul and seven more Tongans jump out. Jeff joins me by the window and we laugh as a sea of Tongans descends on our small home. Enormous men single-handedly hoist bookcases onto their backs. Teenagers carry boxes, teasing one another as they pass on the stairs. Peseti's wife vacuums each room as it's emptied, shooing the younger children away from areas already cleaned. By the time Liz arrives with pizza and sodas for lunch, the entirety of our possessions is crammed into the back of the U-Haul, a good five hours ahead of schedule. Peseti and his cousin decide to leave for Boulder in the rental truck right after lunch, while we spend our last night in San Francisco at Katherine's home across the street. Early the next morning, we begin the eighteen-hour drive—Jeff, Spike, and my godson Chris in one of the SUVs; Vi, Clare, and me in the other.

Two days later, thoroughly exhausted and standing under a mantle of darkness and distant stars, I bounce Clare on my hip and stare in awe at our new home in Boulder. Then we drive the two minutes to Mom and John's home, where we crash for the evening. The following morning, our posse awakens to the smell of coffee and bagels. Peseti and his cousin are well rested, having arrived a day ahead of us. After breakfast, we all pile into our SUVs and drive back to our home less than a quarter-mile away. My body is aching, joints sore from the intensity of the two-day drive. Jeff pulls a chair from the U-Haul and sets it up in the driveway.

"Sit," he says. "Your job is to direct us. Just tell us where things go as we carry them past you."

Our property abuts the trailhead leading to Wonderland Lake, clearly a popular route, judging from the number of people who stroll by wearing hiking boots and wide-brimmed sun hats. I imagine their conversations with one another once they're out of earshot, trying to figure out the story behind the new neighbor with the *Phantom of the Opera* hairdo who's perched on an office chair, barking orders at three large men while pointing with her cane.

Several weeks after our arrival in Boulder, I realize that with less than twenty percent of my hair left, comb-overs and pony-tails have lost their effectiveness. People now look at me with pity. And I don't want pity. I want control.

One day, after swimming at a public pool in Boulder, I ten-tatively approach an attractive twenty-something woman I've seen here before. She has a beautiful confident smile and a closely shaven head.

"Excuse me," I say, "Could you tell me who does your hair?" Her gaze goes directly to my scraggly scalp and she knows I'm not being sarcastic.

"Save yourself some money," she says. "Ten bucks at Wal-green's will get you your own electric shears. That's what I did."

"Thanks," I say and walk away.

"Hey," she calls after me. "You're going to love it. One shaved head and you'll never want hair again!" Feeling calm, even ex-cited, about the idea of proactively removing what remains of my once thick mane, I stop at a pharmacy on the drive home and purchase electric shears.

Tim and Dede and the kids arrive from southern California for a visit several days later. "Since you didn't get my bike," I say to my brother, "the least I can do is give you the honor of shaving my head." He gladly accepts and launches into his im-personation of a hairstylist to the stars, speaking with a goofy French accent. Jeff, Vi, Mom, and John all snicker nervously in that *better you than me* way as they encircle my chair on the back deck. Tim warms up the crowd by telling bad jokes and revving the shears. Dede says she can't watch, and I see tears in her eyes as she turns to go inside. My nieces and nephew—ages eight, six, and five—chant, "Shave it! Shave it! Shave it!" and squeal with glee as Tim makes the first pass across my head. I see strands of hair fall to the ground and think, *Piece of cake*. After Tim makes a few more maneuvers with the shears, my family erupts in laughter. Tim hands me a mirror and I see that he's given me a Mohawk.

"Asshole," I say, much to the delight of his children. Tim resumes his hairstylist duties and minutes later, I run my hand across a smooth scalp.

"Feels good," I say, admiring my new look in the mirror.

"Aunt Wa?" says my six-year-old niece.

"Yes, Andie?"

"I don't think you should've shaved it after all."

33

I LOVE THE FEELING of pulling my body through the water one stroke at a time. I'm much slower than most of the swimmers here, so I always try to score a whole lane for myself. When forced to share, I prefer to split the lane rather than circle because I don't like keeping track of someone else's movements as they advance on me, then pass. My body is still quite tender even now, six months after my hospital discharge. It's not worth the risk of being inadvertently kicked or sideswiped, so I keep to myself in the pool.

Jeff thinks swimming laps is boring, but to me it's a form of motile meditation. All that repetitive back and forth has a mesmerizing effect. I use pithy rhymes as if they're mantras to track my laps. *One, one, this is fun,* I repeat over and over in my head as I swim down the lane the first time. *Two, two, look what I can do,* on the return. Seven and eight are my favorites. *Seven, seven, almost went to heaven. Eight, eight, but now I feel great!* And ten always makes me want to smile, even with my face submerged in chlorinated water. *Ten, ten, let's not do that again.* After twelve, I mentally tally one unit, an exercise measurement I learned years ago at Pepsi's corporate gym. Then I start the series again. Six units equal a mile, and that's exactly what I've just completed, a whole mile. It took me over an hour, slow by any real swimmer's standards. But to me, it's no less than an Olympian feat.

According to my husband, rebuilding my body is my "job" for the foreseeable future. I spend hours each day at the North Boulder Recreation Center, now that autumn has come and all the outdoor public pools are closed until next summer. We've lived here only a couple of months and already I can imagine no other place on earth I'd want to call home. The lifestyle is slower and more relaxed than it is in the major urban areas where I've lived. Makeup is optional, boob jobs unheard of. Many of Boulder's inhabitants rely on hiking, biking, rock climbing, swimming, and skiing to enhance their looks. Others don't even concern themselves with what's considered attractive by mainstream standards, creating a style uniquely their own. Cat Man, as I've nicknamed him, has his entire face tattooed with whiskers and a cute little feline nose. Goth Guy regularly wears four-inch platform boots, their black patent-leather sides rising up to his thighs. And the other day, while I was walking on the Pearl Street pedestrian mall with Clare in the stroller, I saw a ten-inch-high, starch-stiff orange Mohawk. Sporting my head of half-inch-long new hair—a look Jeff has dubbed Eddie Munster—I fit right in.

After my workout, I go home to await the arrival of my cousin, in from England for a multicity vacation to visit family and friends. When Mia and her British naval husband, John, arrive, Jeff and I get them situated in the guest room and show them around our new home. We hear the stirrings of Clare over the baby monitor, so we all move to the nursery to introduce them to their new first cousin once removed.

As Mia bounces Clare on her hip, I recall the discussion we had less than a month before I became pregnant. I was in the middle of my six-week backpacking trip through France and Italy when I received a last-minute invitation from Mia to join her in Spain the following week. John's ship was scheduled to dock in Barcelona for a reprieve from its mission in the Balkans, and the Royal British Navy had granted him a weekend furlough. The three of us gorged on a vegetarian picnic—four different cheeses, freshly baked bread, tomato and avocado slices, olives and cornichons, pistachios, cherries, and two bottles of wine—in the famous Parc Güell, designed and built by Antoni Gaudi in the early 1900s. After lunch we rested in the shade of a pine tree, our backs on the ground and our feet propped up on the trunk of the tree, and talked about life. The subject of children came up, and Mia, ten years my junior, told me that she'd recently been diagnosed with polycystic ovary syndrome. Although they planned to start a family when John's six-month assignment at sea ended, they were uncertain about her ability to conceive.

"What about you?" Mia asked.

"I'll probably be one of those forty-something first-time moms," I said.

"Right," she said. "You know, you're not getting any younger. You might want to get on with it."

"No, we're not ready. Well, Jeff's definitely not ready, and I'm not sure if I'm ready."

"But you're what, thirty-seven, thirty-eight now?"

"Thirty-seven."

"Did you ever consider that when you two finally *are* ready, it might not be physically possible?"

"Look, I just *know* there's a little girl named Clare coming into my life someday. I trust my intuition."

"I prefer to trust science."

"You really ought to get more in touch with your psychic side, Mia."

"And you ought to get more in touch with reality!" We both laughed and moved on to a new topic.

Three weeks later, I was pregnant without even trying. And now, a little over a year later, Mia and John *are* trying, with great difficulty, and I wonder if my cousin is okay being around my happy little family. But I don't ask, am still not ready to have conversations that probe too deeply into the emotions of motherhood, mine or Mia's. I see no obvious signs of sadness as she coos at my baby girl.

That evening, we linger at the dinner table talking of old times. Inevitably, the conversation shifts to yet another rehashing of my close call, with Jeff adding more depth to the story already shared through e-mails and Mia peppering him with questions. He fetches the Sick Photos, as we call them, and passes them around the table over dessert. Between bites of shortbread cookies and sips of herbal tea, John and Mia grimace at images of a bruised and jaundiced body, the dazed look of encephalopathy, a bloated postsurgical belly. This routine has become a regular occurrence when we reconnect with friends for the first time since my hospitalization. Like us, they seem to have a need to talk through their own experience of my illness, the threat of death having permeated their psyches as much as it did ours. And like us, it is the retelling of the story that serves to heal, to shake off the trauma and regain equilibrium.

"I felt so helpless while you were sick," Mia says. "With the time change from California to England, I was always reading Tim's e-mail updates a day later than when things were happening. I wish I could've been more helpful, more hands-on."

"No worries, cuz," I say. "All's well that ends well." And I really believe that, as I sit at the candlelit table with people I adore.

The next day our home takes on the feeling of a hotel as Joey, an old friend from my publishing days, arrives for a one-night layover. We settle him in Clare's room, having already put the portable crib in the master bedroom. An hour later, Jeff leaves for a business trip, his first since our move to Boulder. He has back-to-back meetings with investment bankers in New York City starting early tomorrow morning, and his flight is scheduled to depart Denver at two this afternoon. A couple of hours later, he calls to tell me there are mechanical issues with the airplane and they still haven't boarded. No estimated departure time has been given, so Jeff will wait at the airport rather than make the one-hour drive back home.

My cousins, friend, and I share an early dinner, then settle by the fireplace with Clare nestled in my lap. I pass around the bag of Halloween candy I purchased for next week's trick-or-treaters and slowly work my way through a handful of Tootsie Rolls as we laugh and talk and, once again, discuss the details of my illness. Jeff calls at eight and tells me they're finally boarding. His flight will land in New York around two in the morning, so he promises to call after his meetings tomorrow, which are scheduled to finish at four.

"Looks like I'm going to get only a few hours of sleep tonight, but once I finish tomorrow, I'm free until eleven the next day," he says. "I'll probably just order room service after my meetings and go right to bed."

By the time I awaken the next morning, the nanny has arrived and Joey has departed. Mia and John and I leave for the gym to get a workout in before shopping at the new mall with Clare. After swimming, I lift weights. I've been slowly rebuilding the muscles in my arms and legs using the resistance machines but have yet to tackle my weak and obliterated abdomen. Today, I decide, I'll add abdominal crunches to my routine. Fueled by my desire to recover at warp speed, I do them on an incline board, slowly curling my head and shoulders up toward my feet while struggling against the pull of gravity. The first few crunches feel awkward, my stomach lurching a bit, but eventually I find my rhythm and perform multiple sets of five, stopping at thirty.

Leaving the gym, we decide to have breakfast at Moe's Bagels. Halfway through my salt bagel with olive-pimento cream cheese, I feel an odd sensation in my gut, as if someone's pulling it inward, right behind my navel. I assume the pain is from eating too much candy last night, so I tug my workout tights down a couple inches under my oversized T-shirt and allow my belly to sit unrestricted on top of the waistband. I take another bite of bagel and again I get an uneasy feeling, this time like an internal pinch that makes me wince.

"You okay?" Mia asks.

"Fine," I say. Another spasm sends me jerking forward.

"You sure you're okay?" she asks.

"Maybe not," I say. "I think I may send you shopping without me this afternoon. I'll stay home and nap with Clare."

The rest of my bagel remains untouched, and John and Mia quickly finish eating theirs. We arrive home as the nanny is packing up her things to leave. Clare is sleeping, so I take a shower with the baby monitor on the bathroom counter, the volume turned up as high as it will go. I spend extra time under the spray of the hot water hoping it will calm my ailing belly, but as I towel off in the bedroom, I find myself jerking forward at the waist more vigorously than before. Mia enters the room to see me grip the bedpost and bend forward, like what I imagine a laboring woman would do.

"I don't think we should leave you here alone," she says.

"No, no," I say, not wanting to hamper her brief visit. "I'll be okay if I just rest."

Moments later I feel another tug from behind my navel, this one more severe than all the previous ones. A loud "ah-AY" escapes my mouth, and I can no longer pretend this is the by-product of Tootsie Rolls or a tight waistband. Mia wonders aloud if I have appendicitis, while I've decided my liver is the culprit and it's about to burst.

"Okay," I say between spastic jerks of what must look like a comical rain dance. "I guess I'm not—AHHH!—well. I think I need to see a doc-AYE!-tor."

Mia leaves to get her husband and I slowly dress myself in sweatpants and a sweatshirt, all the while mapping out a plan in my mind. Normally, I'd call my parents for help with babysitting and transportation, but they're visiting my brother's family in California and won't be home until tonight. I have no friends in Boulder yet, only acquaintances, and none that I'd feel comfortable calling. My cousins return and we discuss the best course of action. Mia will stay behind with Clare while her husband and I go to the emergency room. John helps me into their rental car and as we pull out of the driveway, I notice a slight look of panic on his face.

"You okay?" I ask, bent over at the waist and trying hard to look more comfortable than I actually am. "You look like you might puke."

"Right," John says. "It's just that Mia will never forgive me if you expire in our hire car. So please don't."

We both laugh and I wince, the cramps worsening by the minute. I sit up and see that we're driving on the left side of the road.

"We're not in England, John."

"Right," he says, maneuvering the car back to the proper lane.

Two miles from home, we pull the car up to the hospital entrance with the sign that reads Urgent Care. John leaves the car in a no-parking zone and helps me inside. I walk, doubled over, my arms wrapped tightly around my waist, and am taken to an examination room without delay. A nurse hands me a hospital gown and promises to get me something for the pain as soon as they figure out what's wrong. Another nurse assumes John is my husband and asks him for help filling out the paperwork.

"Date of birth?" she asks.

"Sorry, dunno," I hear John reply, and I look up to see an incredulous expression on the nurse's face.

I ask John to find the number for Jeff's hotel in New York and dial it for me. He agrees and steps into the hallway with my cell phone so I can change into my hospital gown. I know Jeff is operating on minimal sleep and I know he'll worry when he hears I'm at the hospital. I also know that he won't forgive me if I don't tell him what's going on. If I leave a voice mail at the hotel instead of on his cell phone, at least he'll be alone when he hears the news, can even pour a drink from the minibar if need be.

There's a knock at the door and John's arm reaches in to hand me the phone as another wave of pain strikes. John has already asked the hotel operator to put the call through to Jeff's room, so moments after putting the phone to my ear, I hear an automated voice telling me to leave my message after the tone.

"Hon-EE!" I blurt out through abdominal convulsions. "Don't wor-EE, but I'm in the EE-mergency room. Not sure what's wrong, but I'll be f-INE. Call my cell!"

I hand the phone back to John as a doctor enters the room. She has me lie on the bed and I try to remain somewhat still while my body continues its involuntary twitching and thrashing with each jolt of abdominal pain. She pushes on different areas of my belly, causing me to yell with each bit of pressure. Turning to a nurse, she orders an immediate X-ray and instructs another nurse to get me some morphine. Within minutes, I'm attached to an IV needle that sends fluids and painkillers coursing through my veins. The first nurse returns moments later, pushing a wheelchair.

"Mrs. Larsen, we need to take you down the hall for X-rays. Are you comfortable sitting, or would you rather lie on a gurney?" she asks.

"Sitting," I say. I ease myself into the wheelchair, but pop back up as if I'd sat on hot coals. The morphine has not yet calmed the spasms and sitting exacerbates the pain.

"I think I'll just walk," I say. The nurse takes my IV pole in one hand and my arm in another and leads me out of the room. Ten steps into our trek to the magnetic imaging department, I feel weak in the knees.

"I think I'm going to pass out," I say, and I sit on a gurney that is parked in the hallway by the nurses' station. "No, actually, I'm going to throw up."

I leap to my feet and look around for a suitable place to vomit. There are two doors in front of me, so I lurch toward the nearest, the nurse and my IV pole close behind. I make it to a small stainless steel sink and eject my bagel and cream cheese all over an array of personalized coffee mugs waiting to be rinsed. The nurse rubs my back as I lean over a large trash can by the sink and vomit more. Someone hands me a smaller trash can so I don't have to bend forward so much, and I throw up in that one as well. I continue heaving even when there is nothing left in my stomach. The convulsions subside and I'm now able to blow my nose and wipe my eyes. Still rubbing my back, the nurse hands me a glass of water. Looking around, I take stock of where I am and realize I've just turned the nurses' coffee-break kitchenette into a scene from *The Exorcist*.

"Sorry," I say, offering an apologetic smile.

"Don't you worry about it," says the nurse. "Happens all the time," she adds, winking.

She asks me to sit in a wheelchair and I oblige, still bent and wincing, but no longer nauseous. Another nurse joins her and the two of them push my wheelchair and IV pole down the hall to X-ray.

"It appears you have a bowel obstruction," says the radiologist, as he clips several large images of my insides up to a lighted panel so we can view them.

"I don't understand," I say.

"Imagine that your intestine is a garden hose. It's as if you have a kink in your hose that's preventing the water from passing through, in this case, waste matter. Things back up and you experience great pain."

"So why did my hose kink?"

"The most common cause is scar tissue. You said you had several surgeries last March?"

"Three in one month."

"That would explain it."

"So how do we *unkink* my garden hose?" I assume there's some sort of drug they'll give me—Drano for intestines—that will clear this up in no time.

"The doctor will discuss treatment with you as soon as she confirms my findings," he says.

I'm wheeled back to the examination room, where John and I wait to meet with the first doctor. The morphine has not fully calmed the storm in my guts, so I'm given another dose. The doctor finally arrives, and I'm hoping she has my little magic unkinking pill with her. She doesn't.

"Mrs. Larsen, we need to prep you for surgery," she says.

What? But this is just a little kink in my garden hose!

Bowel obstructions are common for those who've had multiple abdominal surgeries, she explains, and they're not to be taken lightly. If the intestines don't manage to relax and unknot themselves within a few hours, usually with the help of morphine, surgery is the only way to unobstruct the bowel.

"You'll meet with your surgeon before the operation and he can answer any other questions," she says. "In the meantime, we need to get you to the hospital."

John and I look at one another with mutually stunned expressions. "The hospital?" I ask. "Where the hell are we now?"

We are, we learn, at an independent urgent-care facility. The hospital, it seems, is right across the street. Just as I'm thinking this situation couldn't get any more absurd, I'm told I must be taken by ambulance to the hospital, less than one hundred yards away. Now relaxed and high on morphine, I'm rather enjoying this sitcom as it unfolds in real time. But the laughter and jokes stop cold the minute I see a nurse enter my room with a thick nasogastric tube in her hand, and I'm flooded with distressing memories of intubation. She tells me the tube is necessary to suction any remaining contents from my stomach.

"I can assure you that one hundred percent of the *contents* from my stomach are currently in the sink of that little room down the hall." I say. "So I won't be needing that."

"Your stomach is still producing fluids and we've got to keep them out of there until after the surgery," she says. Her demeanor suggests that I won't be bargaining my way out of this medical protocol, so I take the plastic tube and suck it into my left nostril, gagging as it slides down my throat into my stomach. She attaches the suction bag to the side of my gurney as two young men with ambulance patches on their jackets enter the room.

At the hospital I'm wheeled into a unit that has none of the high-tech, fast-paced feeling of the intensive care unit from last spring. It's more relaxed and seems almost like a clean but low-end hotel, with its requisite tacky wall art and vinyl-covered furniture. I have a view of the Rocky Mountains from my window, and unlike my experience with encephalopathy in San Francisco, this time the mountains are real. Hard plastic nasal tube aside, I'm feeling more at ease now. Even the probability of surgery no longer bothers me, though I recognize that this sense of peace is most likely morphine-induced. My cell phone rings and Jeff's number appears on the display panel.

"Hey, Jeffy," I say, my mellow voice reflecting my drugged state of mind.

"Oh god, honey. Are you okay?" he pleads. "What happened?"

"I'm fine now. Morphine is my friend."

Even sedated, I can tell Jeff has come unglued by the news of my rehospitalization. I fill him in on what I know so far: that surgery is probable, that the surgeon's name is Dr. Johs, that I'll get to meet him as soon as he gets out of his other surgeries, and that I can expect these bowel obstructions to plague me indefinitely because of all the scar tissue in my abdomen. He sounds awful, like he's been crying. He tells me he got only two hours of sleep last night and was bone weary when he returned to his hotel in hopes of having a quick meal and going straight to bed. Seeing the blinking red light on the hotel telephone, he assumed it was a message from me, and finally trusting that our happy outcome to my illness is real, he neither panicked nor worried. But when he heard my message, listened to my voice lurch with each jolt of pain, he reacted in a way I've never witnessed. He threw things. The hotel phone, his Palm Pilot, his briefcase—they all hit the far wall of his hotel room. Then he sat on the side of the bed with his head in his hands until he had calmed himself enough to recover his cell phone and dial my number.

"I'm catching the next flight home," Jeff says. "I promise I'll come straight to the hospital."

"And I promise I won't croak on you," I say. I'm laughing, but even through the haze of morphine I can tell that Jeff isn't.

"Honey?" he says quietly. "I love you. You know that, right?"

"Yes," I say. "I know that beyond a shadow of a doubt. And I love you, too."

We're both quiet. I suspect that Jeff's mind has returned to that place where he was forced to consider losing me while I was in the ICU, and that makes my own thoughts return to the fatal traffic accident I narrowly escaped two weeks before Clare's birth.

"Jeff? Please don't worry," I say. "Remember, it's not my time."

It's early evening when I finally meet the surgeon. Wearing hiking shorts and sandals, Dr. Johs strides into my room, clipboard in hand. He perfectly fits my preconceived notion of a Boulder doctor and I like him immediately.

"Sorry for not getting to you sooner," he says. "Been a pretty full day in the OR."

Pulling a chair up to my bed, he sits eye level with me, and I make a mental note that he gets bonus points for bedside manner. "I'm Stephen," he says, extending his right hand. First-name basis? More points.

He flips through my medical chart, offering an occasional *hmm* or *aha*. "How're you feeling now?" he asks.

"Pretty good," I say. "Other than the fact that I feel like I have a pencil shoved up my nose." My abdomen has relaxed, but the nasogastric tube is still irritating my head and throat. He smiles knowingly.

"How long's it been since your last bout of abdominal pain?"

"Over two hours."

This is a good sign that surgery may not be necessary after all, he explains. I'll have to remain under observation in the hospital for several days, but for now, he's cancelling the operation until further notice.

"That's great," I say. "There's one more thing, though. This nose tube is killing me. There's almost nothing in the drainage bag. Can we *please* remove this godforsaken thing if I promise not to whine if it needs to be reinserted later?"

I watch his face as he contemplates my request. He's either a stellar actor, or he's taking me seriously as a collaborator in my own care.

"Sure," he says. And with that one simple word, Dr. Johs—Stephen—has become my new best friend.

After the consultation, I send John home to be with his wife and my baby. I close my eyes to rest, knowing Jeff will be here in a few hours.

"Oh, for Christ's sake! Haven't you put all of us through enough already?"

Even sedated, I recognize that sarcasm and laughter as belonging to Mom. I open my eyes as she and my stepdad walk into my room. They sit in chairs at the foot of the bed, and she tells me that Mia filled them in on my medical emergency when Mom phoned from the Denver airport.

"I've already called all your siblings," she says. "Tim said to give you a message."

"What's that?" I ask.

"He says to hurry up and die already because no one in the family can take any more of the mental anguish of having you in the hospital." We both laugh. My family's propensity for dark humor has always been our greatest coping mechanism.

"I'm surprised he didn't call dibs on my bike."

"He did!"

Three days later, I'm released from the hospital with a renewed commitment to take my recovery more seriously.

34

"You want to put a needle in my *tweeter*?" I ask, not quite sure I heard her right.

I'm lying on the table midway through my second acupuncture session with my new doctor of Oriental medicine, and she looks at me with an expression that is both humoring and perplexed. I'm no stranger to this healing practice, and I've had acupuncture needles in my head, face, and toes before, but never in my crotch. I'd always assumed that was the off-limits zone. Apparently not.

"If your perineum is the same as a tweeter, then yes, I want to put a needle in your tweeter," she says, offering a forced chuckle.

I don't bother explaining the origin of the term tweeter, which Jeff and I made up years ago when Spike would stand at the window and bark incessantly at the squirrels on our back patio. We couldn't help but notice how silly she looked, her sphincter popping away from her backside with each bark, like the woofer on a stereo speaker blasted at full volume. "Spike, be careful or you'll blow your woofer," Jeff always told her. Somehow, jokes about Spike's "woofer" led to the creation of the corresponding term "tweeter," and over the years it stuck.

"I know it's a bit invasive, so the decision is yours," she says. "This is a very powerful acupuncture point, almost like the reset button on a computer. Given all you've been through, it could be quite beneficial to your recovery."

"Why not?" I say, though I can think of at least five good reasons why not.

She asks me to slip off my slacks and underpants, which I do, feeling no modesty whatsoever. She instructs me to lie on my back and pull my knees to my chest, and when she hands me a tissue to "cover myself," as she says, I burst out laughing.

"You're kidding, right?"

Her expression tells me she's not, so I take the tissue and arrange it over my pubic hair.

"Now remember, this will be brief, but I'll need to stimulate the acupuncture point before I remove the needle," she says. Stimulate, I've learned, is acupuncture code for *twist the needle around until the patient squirms and/or yells with pain.*

Why did I agree to this again? As soon as I think these words, the answer surfaces: because I want my body back, free of constant joint pain, bowel obstructions, and half of each day given over to sleep. I want the physical strength to play with and care for my baby girl, to be able to walk across a room with her in my arms and know that I won't drop her, as I've already done twice when my legs simply gave out beneath me. I want recovery in the worst way and I'm willing to try anything to get there. So far, my repertoire of healing approaches includes both mainstream and alternative: biweekly physical therapy sessions; concoctions of kale, carrots, apples, cucumbers, lemons, garlic, and wheatgrass made with my new juicer; ozone therapy, in which I sit with my head sticking out of a one-person sauna while ozone seeps into my pores; a special alkalizing powder I mix with rice milk each morning. And this.

As the acupuncturist inserts the needle in my perineum, I squelch the desire to leap from the table and run for my car, pants or no pants. Between muffled groans, I remind myself that I've survived not one, but two, liver biopsies through the neck. *You can handle this,* I tell myself. Thirty seconds later, she removes the needle and I let out an audible sigh of relief.

"Sorry, I know that must've been difficult," she says.

"Sure beats a transjugular liver biopsy," I say. Again, I get the amused but confused look.

"A what?"

"A liver biopsy through the neck. I've had two done that way because my body was too bloated to do them through my belly."

"Sounds awful."

"It was. But now anytime something bad happens, I ask myself if it's worse than a transjugular liver biopsy. If it isn't, I quit whining. If it is, I get to gripe all I want."

"Hmm," she says, and I can't tell if she approves of the attitude adjustment system I've devised. She takes my pulse in three different locations around my wrist and furrows her brow.

"I'm afraid I didn't quite get the right point," she says, offering me an apologetic look. "You willing to try again?"

Oh, good lord.

"Sure," I say. So again, she plunges a needle into my perineum and again I suppress the urge to yell or flee or both. When she tells me a second time that she missed the point, for some reason I can't fathom, I agree to another try.

"Third time's a charm," she says after testing my pulse points afterward. I put my clothes on and write her a check for the session, which I know my insurance company won't cover. After recently learning that my medical bill totaled roughly $750,000, I don't begrudge the company its lack of alternative treatment coverage. The acupuncturist has already estimated that I'll require a series of twelve weekly sessions, but despite my proven ability to take a needle in the tweeter, I never return.

My recovery process has been a comedic, and somewhat costly, lesson in trial and error. During my last week in the hospital after Clare's birth eight months ago, I'd asked several of my doctors if they had any suggestions for me once I left their care. I received but one recommendation: Don't drink any alcohol for a year. *No shit*, I remember thinking. It didn't seem adequate advice for someone whose body was decimated, every major organ save my heart having been pushed to the brink. One nurse—a favorite—decided to break with protocol and give me advice behind the doctors' backs. Looking over her shoulder as if to ensure no one was listening, she suggested I pick up a comprehensive nutrition book by a popular alternative-healing author. She also suggested that I incorporate various supplements and foods rich in antioxidants into my diet. And some day, she said, when I felt strong enough, it would be good for me to undertake an extensive "liver cleanse" program. I had no idea what she was talking about, but I took notes and thanked her profusely.

Launching my recovery felt like being sent on a journey but given no map. I've since learned that no map exists for what I survived, so I venture off in one direction or another based on input from an array of people, like asking for directions in a tourist town, never quite sure of the accuracy of the responses. Even the MDs I see in Boulder can't seem to agree on my prognosis for recovery. One believes I have celiac disease and tells me to give up wheat forever, while another tests me for neurological disorders. A third doctor tells me to accept that I'll never heal completely, that I "should be dead," and as such, should be happy with the physically limited body I now have. One physician, whom I quickly come to adore, actually takes the time to read through my full medical record and then spends two hours with me on an intake visit. Unfortunately, pressure from insurance companies to spend an average of ten minutes or less with each patient pushes his principles to the brink, and shortly after I begin seeing him, he closes his practice.

Given my recent hospitalization for the bowel obstruction, I decide it's time to give that liver cleanse a try. Sitting on an old wicker stool in the book section of a local organic grocer, I peruse all the books with the word "cleanse" in their titles. I buy the one that outlines a two-week fasting program designed to detoxify my liver. The next day I return to the same store and stock up on everything I'll need for the program: Epsom salts, probiotics, vegetables to make a cleansing broth, lemons, olive oil, herbal teas, and more vitamins than I thought possible for one person to ingest. I'd always equated fasting with saving money, but I leave the store having spent more than $300 on my supplies.

The afternoon is spent boiling vegetables: kale, spinach, broccoli, sweet potatoes, carrots, cauliflower, nori and dulse seaweed, white and green onions. Straining the soup, I fill pitcher after pitcher with my first batch of "cleansing broth" and toss a few of the soggy vegetables into Spike's bowl. She eyes them suspiciously, sniffs around the bowl a bit, and walks away. Not a good sign if even the dog doesn't show interest.

Propping my cleanse book open on the kitchen counter, I write up the schedule of what vitamin is to be taken when, what time I'm to brew the tea, when I'm to have a cup of broth for my meals. Other than dabbling with a few fad diets in college when weight loss was the last thing I needed, I've never put myself on a regimented food plan, let alone a liver-detox program. Jeff walks into the kitchen and surveys the scene.

"Wow. Looks like a lot of work for a fast," he says.

"It is. And remember, I don't want you tempting me with any real food. I'm going to try to make it at least ten days," I tell him.

"Hey, I'll support whatever helps you recover." He opens the refrigerator and scans the shelves, all relatively naked in preparation for my program launch tomorrow.

"What do you want for dinner?" Jeff asks.

"Pizza," I say. "Extra cheese."

The next morning I awaken, take my warm water with freshly squeezed lemon juice and a vitamin C. Half an hour later, I drink herbal tea. More vitamins. *Really wish I could have a bagel.* More tea. Choke down two tablespoons of olive oil mixed with the juice of half a lemon. Famished, I check the time. Ten thirty.

How the hell am I going to make it ten full days? More vitamins. At eleven, I get to have my first cup of warm cleansing broth. I heat the brownish water, pour it into a thick mug, and take a sip. It's so weak in flavor I can barely drink half the cup. As I pour the rest down the drain, reasons this fast is a stupid idea bombard my mind. Maybe my liver's not so bad off after all. Food is necessary. Who drinks olive oil anyway?

"How's the cleanse going so far?" asks our nanny, Jean, as she bounces my baby on her hip.

"Sucks," I say, lifting Clare from her arms.

Jean warms a bottle and hands it to me. As Clare slurps down her meal, I find myself coveting her culinary pleasure. All these months later, it still makes me laugh to watch her pump her arms in joy over eight ounces of soy formula. Eating is supposed to be fun, I think. Not work. When Clare finishes, Jean takes her upstairs for a diaper change before her nap. I open the refrigerator, then the freezer, looking, wishing.

"Screw it," I mutter under my breath, as I toss a bag of frozen tortellini onto the countertop. I pull three pans from beneath the stove and boil water for the pasta. In a smaller saucepan, I melt butter, add flour, milk, minced garlic, and parmesan cheese—all staples that haven't been purged from our kitchen for my cleanse. Stirring my thickening concoction, I simultaneously pull fresh spinach from the refrigerator and begin sautéing it in yet another pan. More butter, more garlic. Ten minutes later, my meal is ready, Clare is asleep, and Jean sets the baby monitor on the kitchen counter before leaving, her half-day shift complete. I pour myself a Coke and take my plate of tortellini Alfredo and spinach to the living room, where I load my worn copy of *It's a Wonderful Life* into the VCR. Less than four hours after launching my ten-day liver cleanse, it's over. Instead, my recovery plan for today will consist of the creamy joy of one of my favorite foods and the saccharine sentimentality of my favorite movie.

35

DURING OUR FIRST THANKSGIVING in Boulder, Liz and her husband come to visit, and over dinner she and Jeff entertain Rick and me with stories of the various doctors they dealt with while I was hospitalized. There is one, Ichabod, whose name dominates the conversation.

"Do you remember those first few days at the second hospital?" Jeff asks Liz. "When that jerk started every sentence with 'Well, if she lives …'."

"Oh god, how could I forget?" Liz says, taking another swig of her cabernet. "Even if you thought her odds were slim, what kind of moron says that—repeatedly, much less—to the patient's spouse?"

"He really said that?" Rick asks.

" 'Well, if she lives. Well, if she lives,'" Jeff says, imitating our least favorite doctor.

"Augh," Liz says, disgusted. "Don't get me started. That guy pissed me off to no end."

If there's one person you don't want to piss off, it's Liz, the quintessential porcupine, whose quills spring into action the minute a threat approaches. I've seen some fairly ferocious responses from my friend over the years toward those she deemed rude or cruel, responses I would never have had the guts to make, but that I've laughed myself silly about afterward. She proceeds to tell us about her interaction with Ichabod during my fifth day in the hospital.

The story goes like this: Ichabod came into my ICU room one night to examine the surgical wounds on my abdomen as I lay comatose in bed and Liz sat quietly in the corner. He pulled the blanket that covered me down to my knees and pulled my hospital gown up to my breasts. When the examination was complete, he promptly turned and left, with no acknowledgment to Liz and no move to return my hospital gown or my bed sheets to their original position. Liz interpreted this as a blatant lack of respect for me, coherent or not, a show of hubris that implied *I'm too busy to be bothered.*

I can picture Liz—tall, thin, and confident, with her steely no-nonsense look—as she calmly set her magazine aside, rose to her feet, and followed Ichabod into the ICU's busy hallway.

"Excuse me," she said, the slight edge in her voice akin to the rattle of a deadly snake before it strikes. Ichabod kept walking away, seemingly unaware that he was being paged. "Excuse me!" she repeated, with a bit more volume.

That got Ichabod's attention. In fact, it got the attention of everyone standing in the hallway. Five or so people turned toward Liz. "Are you finished examining my friend?" Liz asked, holding Ichabod's gaze so there would be no mistaking the target of her inquisition. "Because if you are, I would appreciate you showing her some respect by putting her hospital gown and blanket back the way they were instead of leaving her exposed as you did."

"You said that?" I ask, interrupting her.

"You're damn right I did!" Liz says, her anger from the interchange still apparent.

"What'd he say?" I ask, laughing at my pal's ballsy attitude.

"Nothing," she replies. "He stared at me like I was nuts. You could tell that all the wide-eyed nurses surrounding him were psyched, though, as if they wanted to yell *Right on! Put that jackass in his place!*"

"I never heard this story," Jeff says, also laughing.

"One of the nurses finally told Ichabod she'd take care of it," Liz continues. "And that jerk just shook his head and walked away from me without a word. But I'll bet he thought twice before disrespecting a patient like that again!" She throws her head back, letting loose a boisterous laugh.

While the story is amusing and provides yet another puzzle piece for my continued understanding of what happened, it also reminds me how lucky I am to have friends like Liz—and Pam and Sabra and every one of my family members, all of whom joined forces and became my personal advocates at the hospital, all day, every day. Who advocates for those without friends or family who live in town or have the resources to fly in from elsewhere? Who makes sure the hospital staff knows more about the patient than her list of medical ailments? That her favorite color is purple. That she's a fighter and is prone to swearing, nothing personal. That she prefers calm music to the background noise of the hospital television. That there's a baby out there who needs this patient to recover, to come home and be her mother.

To say that I am grateful is an understatement. But gratitude wasn't something that permeated my being the minute I regained consciousness in the hospital, despite what made-for-television medical dramas would have us believe. It didn't happen when I took my first steps, or when I left the hospital, or even when I held my baby girl for the first time after she came home to live with us at two months old. For me, gratitude was like a gentle river, patiently cascading over and around me, finding the small cracks in the hardened shell that helped me focus on the physical challenges of my situation without distraction from the emotional aftershocks of trauma. Aided by details of my story that others remember and share with me, gratitude probes and penetrates until it saturates my understanding of the near-fatal experience, until there is so much of it I don't know how to begin expressing it.

Between hospital stories, we are quiet, as if waiting for another memory to surface. Liz is the first to break the silence. "Remember when Clare was just a few days old and she stopped breathing?"

"What!" I scream. "I never heard this!"

"Oh god, I'd forgotten about that," Jeff says. "Or maybe I blocked it from my memory."

"You were a complete train wreck at that point," Liz says to me. "I decided to take a break from all the sadness of your situation and go see Clare, who was referred to as the 'boarder baby' down in the nursery."

"Boarder baby?" I ask.

"She was 'boarding' at the hospital at that point because she no longer needed their care," Jeff says. "But since there was no one at home, the pediatrician fudged her medical records so she could stay at the hospital with all of us."

"Anyway, I walked down to the nursery and there was a crowd of medical people surrounding Clare's bassinet," Liz says. "When things finally calmed down, they told me that she'd stopped breathing."

"Like we needed one more emergency," Jeff says, shaking his head and reaching for the wine bottle.

"Luckily, one of the nurses on duty happened to be walking past her crib and noticed that she was turning blue," Liz continues. "They got her breathing again pretty quickly, but damn."

"What caused it?" I ask.

"They never figured it out," Liz says. "Chalked it up to an unexplainable SIDS moment."

Sudden Infant Death Syndrome? Clare?

I sit, incredulous, with this latest bit of information, another of the puzzle pieces being handed to me by those who know more about my story than I do. And then, the gratitude. How amazing that Clare was in the care of medical professionals when it *did* happen. How fortuitous that the pediatrician had

faked the records a bit, allowing her to stay at the hospital longer than deemed necessary by the insurance company. And how
absolutely unimaginable to think that the little girl, almost nine
months old and sleeping soundly upstairs, might not have been
in my life today. Grateful doesn't begin to describe it.

Shortly after Liz and Rick's visit, Mom hands me her typed
notes, titled Lauren's Log, and I learn even more remarkable
details of my story, of the numerous times my body seemed
to check out, followed by inexplicable comebacks. When I get
to the part where Mom whispers in my ear about how strong
Capricorns are, I'm stunned. Grabbing the phone, I call her and
skip any greeting.

"How many times in the hospital did you talk to me about
Capricorns being strong and capable of overcoming great obstacles?" I demand more than ask.

"Just that once, when you were comatose. Augh," she says as
if reliving the moment. "You looked god-awful, and you didn't
hear a word I said."

"But I did!" I yell. "I remember that conversation like it was
yesterday! Only I didn't realize I was comatose or that I wasn't
actually speaking myself. But I remember every single word you
said to me!"

"Holy shit," Mom says.

"No shit, holy shit," I say. We laugh and say our goodbyes so
I can continue reading.

My reaction shifts from sadness to amazement with each
page I turn. The details of suffering that run throughout Lauren's Log are offset by example after example of kindness and
decency and compassion, and this opens up more cracks, more
gratitude flowing to and from the core of my soul. I read about
people who don't even know me hosting blood drives in my
honor, and others, also strangers, initiating prayer chains for
me. But what stands out the most are all the instances of hu-

manity repeatedly displayed by the nurses at both hospitals: in Labor & Delivery, the ICU, the Transitional ICU, and finally, Critical Care. Even after I was released from their care, several of my nurses would regularly visit me in my new unit, bringing their lunches with them or spending a ten-minute coffee break in my room. By the time I finish reading all forty-seven pages of Lauren's Log, I'm speechless. What to do with all this gratitude? I know I want do something to say thank you. To whom, I don't know. There are so many to thank.

A few days later, it occurs to me what a consequential role my nurses played, not only in my care, but also in the care of my husband and family. I pick up the phone and call one of my favorite nurses, Carol Abrahams, who regularly took the shuttle across town to see me after I was transferred from the hospital where she worked to the main campus. I had no memory of her from the first hospital, but a friendship blossomed during our visits at the second.

"I want to launch a give-back campaign," I tell Carol over the phone. "I want to say thank you by running a marathon and raising money for a cause." Carol listens quietly, and doesn't even laugh when I say the word *marathon*. "I want nursing to be that cause."

"That's very sweet," she says, when I finally pause. "But the people you really ought to thank are at the blood center. That was an awful lot of blood you went through."

"That much?" I ask.

"Let's just say you single-handedly created a blood shortage in San Francisco while you were sick."

Days later, with Carol's help, I'm on the phone with a woman named Deb from Blood Centers of the Pacific. I explain my desire to do something, speaking quickly and breathlessly, as if to get all the words out before she thinks me a nutcase and hangs up. She gives me the name of Barb at the regional office in Phoenix. I call her, and she gives me the name and number of their national affiliate in Washington, D.C. I pick up the phone and dial the number for America's Blood Centers.

"Jim MacPherson," the voice on the other end of the line says. I immediately launch into my *I-almost-died-and-I'm-so-grateful-to-be-alive-that-I-want-to-give-back* spiel, which I've perfected during my earlier calls. I go on and on, as if my very existence depends on this man's willingness to accept my offer to fund-raise for his organization. Finally, I stop talking to take a breath.

"What is it you want?" Jim says, not unkindly, but clearly perplexed about my agenda.

"Your mailing address," I say. "And who the checks ought to be made out to." He laughs and gives me both.

Several months later, on Clare's first birthday, I launch my campaign, *2001: A Blood Odyssey*, by mailing more than six hundred letters to friends, family members, and former colleagues. I tell people my story and ask them to sponsor me in the New York City Marathon next November by giving blood or money, both if they're so inclined.

Then I do something I haven't done since the early months of my pregnancy. I lace up my running shoes, and with Clare strapped into the purple baby jogger, I make my way down the driveway and onto Northstar Court, to Wonderland Hill Drive, Linden Avenue, and then Fourth Street, clinging to the jogger for support. I wobble along the route to Pearl Street, just as I had visualized while still learning to walk again. Only slower. Much slower.

My training gains momentum over the following weeks, as does my campaign. The original letter is forwarded to other people, some of whom I know, but most total strangers. A journalist from my hometown in New Jersey gets a copy, and although my family moved from the area when I was eighteen, soon there's an article about my marathon campaign in the local paper. I begin hearing from the unlikeliest of people: my first boyfriend, my high school English teacher, even the cute guy in my eleventh grade art class on whom I once had a wicked crush. Reply forms and notes of encouragement start arriving in the mail, and I find myself waiting for the mailman to show up each day so I can get my daily dose of what I can only describe as love. Many people take my suggestion to donate $5 for each mile and send checks for $131. Many more simply send what they can—$5, $10. Others send a commitment to donate blood, some for the first time ever.

People share with me their own stories of blood transfusion, how it saved their child's life or why they began donating blood years ago. The wife of Jeff's former business partner writes that she's always been afraid of needles, so she took a friend along to hold her hand while she made her first blood donation the previous week. Another friend says that his fear of needles is so great that he can't donate blood. Instead, he sends a check for $200. A former Pepsi colleague writes that her sister recently died of cancer, but that she'd been given an extra year of life thanks to regular blood transfusions. And a former publishing colleague returns my reply card with a simple message. *This is a stupid idea*, she writes next to my bold declaration to run a marathon. Then she proceeds to list all the physiological reasons why it's too soon to put my body through such a challenge. (Weeks after the marathon, she sends me another simple message: *I still think it was a stupid idea*, her card reads, *but congratulations anyway.* Included in her envelope is a donation for $2,600, my largest to date.)

Two months after launching my campaign, I board a plane to San Francisco with Jeff and Clare to speak at the annual recognition luncheon hosted by Blood Centers of the Pacific. This is the first time I'll be speaking to a large audience in over three years. There was a time when, working as a marketing professional, I couldn't wait for the national sales meetings each year because it was a chance to get on stage and be a ham. I took full advantage of my counterparts' more traditional presentations to stand out with my own style. I'd publicly sung and danced to disco tunes, written and performed rap lyrics, driven a Mountain Dew van down the center aisle of a conference hall, and even snuck Spike into a swanky hotel through a fire exit so I could include her in a satirical skit I'd written. I was as comfortable speaking to five hundred people as I was to five, but on the day of the blood center event, I spend nearly an hour in the restroom with stress-induced diarrhea.

When the time comes for me to give my talk, Jeff knocks on the bathroom door and coaxes me back to the banquet room, where nearly four hundred people sit eating dessert and drinking coffee. The blood center's director of public relations, Lisa Bloch, introduces me and I make my way to the microphone. *Louder!* I hear from the back of the room after barely getting my first words out. I look at Jeff, sitting nearby with Clare and Sabra. He nods, as if willing me to be calm, to enjoy the spotlight. *You can do it,* he says with his eyes.

Five minutes into my talk, I realize that the clinking of silverware and the side conversations have ceased, that I have the full attention of everyone in the room. As I tell my story, I notice how good it feels to share the details, both painful and joyful, with this group of strangers who are starting to feel like friends. I'm only eight pages into my twelve pages of notes when I notice Lisa standing off to the side, inching closer and closer to the podium, a bouquet of flowers in her arms—my signal to wrap it up. But like a marathon therapy session, my verbal catharsis continues for a full half hour past the allotted time, my need to retell the entire story, as I now know it, superseding my desire to be respectful of the event schedule. When I finally offer my closing remarks to this room full of San Francisco's most loyal blood donors, they break out in a standing ovation, not only for my survival of the illness, I suspect, but for their own survival of my long-windedness. As they crowd me with hugs and pats on the back, I openly weep with a year's worth of pent-up gratitude.

36

FIVE MONTHS INTO MY MARATHON TRAINING, I receive a phone call at home from my Pilates instructor. More of a physical therapist, she's been helping me address some of the challenges of preparing my still-recovering body for a 26-mile race. She asks me if I own an SUV, and I wonder what connection that could possibly have to my surviving the impending marathon. When I tell her yes, she asks me if I'd be willing to drive some refugees to a picnic that weekend. I tell her sure, and after we say goodbye, I call down to Jeff in his home office.

"Honey? Where's Sudan?"

That Saturday, Jeff, Clare, and I drive to a dilapidated rental home on the outskirts of Denver and introduce ourselves to several tall dark men, all of whom appear to be in their late teens and early twenties. With Clare sandwiched between several of them, we drive into the mountains above Boulder to a wooded campground where thirty or so other refugees—all recent arrivals to the U.S.—and an equal number of Americans are gathered. Together, we roast hot dogs and hamburgers and play tag football, and when the games and food are exhausted, we sit in small groups throughout the picnic area and hear the refugees' stories.

Without apparent emotion, these gentle young men known as the Lost Boys of Sudan calmly tell us how they were at school or tending cattle when government-backed raiders attacked their villages, raping women and girls, capturing some as slaves, and killing men, women, and children who were unable to escape. We hear in horrifying detail how they ran from aerial bombings and the gunfire of soldiers. Fleeing into the bush and separated from their families, these boys—ages five to twelve at the time—wandered in no apparent direction, meeting up with other small groups of boys from nearby villages that had been raided as well. They walked and walked, at times so hungry they ate mud and so thirsty they drank their own urine. They walked every day for months until they made it to a refugee camp in Ethiopia, where they remained for a year until civil war broke out. Commanded to leave the country at gunpoint, many were shot by soldiers even as they were obeying the order to evacuate. Others were forced to keep swimming across the Nile despite the desperate cries of their friends who were unable to swim or who'd been caught in the jaws of a crocodile. And at night, when they slept on the ground in a tight cluster, the boys at the outermost edge of the group would creep over sleeping bodies to get closer to the center. This process would continue until dawn, each boy hoping to avoid the inevitable attack of a hungry lion during the night.

The details of their stories are so shocking and so far removed from my own experience that at times I have to step away and take a moment to connect with the beauty of the alpine trees that surround us or simply stroll hand in hand with my little girl before returning to the group to hear more.

By the time the Lost Boys made it to another refugee camp in Kenya, they had walked more than 1,000 miles. Of the estimated 30,000 boys who had fled their war-ravaged villages during the genocide attacks throughout southern Sudan, roughly half survived the journey. They then spent a decade living in the harsh conditions of the camps, seeking whatever education they could, playing soccer with balls that were sometimes no more than a wad of trash taped together, and continually trying to get word about family members: who had survived, who hadn't. Many of our new young friends are still uncertain as to the fate of their parents and siblings. Coming to the U.S. weeks earlier, and with no formal documents to determine their dates of birth, they were all assigned the generic birthday of January 1 by the immigration service. Shortly after their arrival, someone from one of the local relief agencies decided to organize a social outing in hopes of garnering more support from people who might help in whatever ways they saw fit.

After leaving the picnic that day, both Jeff and I feel that another new adventure in our lives has just begun. Many other local residents who attended apparently feel the same way, and soon a whole group of us from Denver and Boulder are e-mailing and organizing and sharing ideas. We decide to each "adopt" a household of Sudanese refugees, and we ask one of the relief agency representatives to help us in making those individual assignments.

Two weeks after the picnic, I strap Clare into her car seat for my first of many drives to Denver to act as a substitute mother to eight guys who are so culturally different I'm a bit overwhelmed. I have no experience with refugees, no understanding of the deep-seated emotional trauma that will surface over time. All I know is this: I am a mother who can't fathom the idea of her own child enduring half of what these young men have, let alone what their less fortunate female counterparts have. So, as a mother, I want to offer my help to these boys. I have no idea what to do, but I'll figure it out as I go. Because that's what we mothers do.

Entering a questionable downtown neighborhood, I find the address, then circle the block several times to determine the safest place to park. Balancing Clare on my hip, I make my way across an unkempt courtyard with more broken glass and trash on the ground than grass. At least three different stereo systems boom music into the quad, and I question the intelligence of bringing my daughter with me on this first excursion. I knock on the door of a run-down ground-level apartment and wonder how best to break the ice. What do you say to a group of young men whose childhoods have been irrevocably lost to war and hate and violence?

Daniel, James, Gabriel, Chuor, Peter, Panther, Abraham, and John all share a cramped two-bedroom apartment that reeks of fetid cooking oil and mildew. One by one, they each shake my hand, their eyes downcast in a Sudanese show of respect. Then they crowd around Clare, smiling broadly and allowing her to grip their fingers or touch their hair. Our brief greetings complete, I scan the room like a mother assessing her child's college dormitory for the first time. One-third of the living area is crammed with used bicycles donated by a local church. A baby's broken high chair and a massive nonworking console television fill another wall. A card table and four mismatched folding chairs, shoved against one of the two shabby couches, serve as the dining area. In each bedroom I find garbage bags overflowing with secondhand clothing, filling what little space remains between the queen-size bed, a twin bed, and the walls. A tiny hall closet is filled with old skis, impractical kitchen appliances, and other assorted items that serve no purpose and claim precious storage space. I sit at the card table and pull pen and paper from my purse to take notes. There is much work to be done and many supplies to procure for these boys, my newly adopted sons.

I ask the guys questions and try piecing together the meaning of their responses, spoken in broken English and with thick Dinka accents. None of them feels comfortable shopping for groceries, they tell me, so all eight of them cram into my SUV and we drive to a nearby Safeway. Unbeknownst to me, the local paper had run a lengthy article about the Lost Boys that morning, so as the guys hover by my side while I push Clare's stroller through the grocery store, strangers tentatively approach us to inquire if these are indeed the young refugees about whom they've read. Greetings and encouraging words are offered, and one woman gives me twenty dollars to help cover the cost of their groceries. We visit the deli section and I ask the man behind the counter if he'll allow them to sample various cheeses and lunchmeats. He does, but the guys' taste buds are so muted from the monotony of eating maize, beans, and sorghum for most of their lives, the only thing they like is the sliced roast beef. We order three pounds of it, and while we wait, Daniel asks me where in the store the live cattle are kept.

A woman behind the bakery counter calls to us, waving. She too read the article that morning and has already cut eight large slices of cake, one for each Lost Boy. As she hands them each a paper plate and plastic fork, they smile and thank her, but after the first bite they turn to me with imploring looks, like toddlers with mouths full of kale. I tell them to follow me and we walk inconspicuously out of the bakery worker's line of vision. I find a trashcan, collect the plates of remaining cake, and throw them all away.

We wander up and down aisles, the Lost Boys pointing at various items and me explaining what each is. John picks up an antiperspirant stick, so I mime putting deodorant under my arms and the guys all nod their understanding. Abraham picks up a box of tampons and asks me what they are, and I stammer, not knowing how to delicately convey their purpose without causing him embarrassment. When I'm finally able to do so, the guys chuckle and playfully punch Abraham's arm, and I sense that underneath all the cultural differences, teenaged boys have more in common than I thought.

Reaching the produce section of the store, the guys ooh and ahh at all the choices. We load bags of potatoes and apples and carrots into the shopping cart, all items I think will agree with their adjusting systems. The produce manager approaches to say hello and asks if there is anything else they'd like.

"Where is the okra, please?" Daniel says to him.

"The what?" the manager replies.

For the next ten minutes, no less than four different Safeway employees are involved in a comical snipe hunt for a vegetable none of them would recognize even if they could locate it. We leave the store with bags of vegetables and rice, beef and chicken, bread in every imaginable form, milk, toothpaste, toilet paper, and sponges. I drop the guys back at their apartment, then begin the trip home to Boulder.

While I drive, it occurs to me how focused I've been on my own healing over the past year. Yet now life has given me the opportunity to focus on someone else's healing, and this alone gives me a greater sense of purpose than anything I'd ever done in my previous career. My body and energy level may still be too depleted to return to work, but I know I have skills that can help these young men. I know I can make a difference in their lives. What I don't yet know—but will soon learn—is how healing it is for me to focus on the healing of another.

The following week Jeff loads the SUV with extra pots, cooking utensils, Tupperware containers, towels, and blankets from our home. Clare and I again drive to Denver, this time with my friend Susanna and her young son following us in their car. We stop at Costco on the way and fill the back of both vehicles with cases of soup, loaves of bread, chicken, beef, lentils, pasta, jumbo tubs of butter, powdered lemonade, and multipacks of soap, shampoo, vitamins, cleaning supplies, and laundry detergent. When we arrive at the Lost Boys' home, I introduce them to "Mom" Susanna—a common term of respect given to the many women who've become involved in helping them. They all pitch in to unload the two cars while Susanna and I empty cupboards and wipe them down before restocking them. As our toddlers suck on sippy cups on the couch, we move through the guys' apartment and help them clean and organize. I direct them to carry broken items that came with this "furnished" apartment to the dumpster, assuring them that they won't get in trouble for doing so. The huge console television and the high chair are the first two items to go. The 1970s-era electric hotdog cooker, skis, a broken clock, and torn baskets are next. We sort through the bags of clothing, and the guys pick out only those items they like enough to wear. The rest go in the back of my SUV for delivery to the nearest Goodwill. Susanna teaches them how to cook pasta with tomato sauce and buttery garlic bread while I show them how to mix the powdered lemonade, and then we all share a simple meal together.

When I return for my next visit, I find the carpet soggy with moisture throughout an entire bedroom and out into the hallway. Daniel explains that the water pipes in the community laundry room next to their apartment burst, flooding their living space, over a week ago. Four at a time, the guys have been taking turns sleeping in the one remaining bedroom. The manager of the complex has ignored their pleas for help, and I'm certain their status as recent immigrants makes it easier for him to put off the repairs. Angered, I get the phone number of the property manager and take out my cell phone. Doing my best impersonation of an attorney, I leave a voice-mail message, threatening to take legal action if the problem isn't remedied immediately. Days later, someone arrives to vacuum the excess water and clean the carpet. Still, I'm angered by the property manager's blatant disregard for those who both live in poverty and have a language barrier. As a country, we've opened our doors to these young men. Individually, however, the response to their arrival ranges from the kindest acts of compassion to the rudest of ignorance.

Weeks later, some of the guys and I return to Safeway, this time to secure job applications. I ask to see the manager and when he arrives, each of the guys shakes his hand and looks him directly in the eye, just like we've practiced. It quickly becomes clear that Peter's six missing front teeth—cut out as a rite of passage when he was five—are going to be an impediment to securing employment, as they cause him to lisp, further hindering his ability to be assertive. That night, I spread the word through e-mail that I need to find a dentist willing to do some pro bono work. A friend of a friend responds, saying that she's a dental hygienist and her boss is willing to help. The first time I see Peter after he's received his new teeth, I barely recognize him. No longer sitting quietly on the sidelines, he begins speaking up, even smiling. And the dentist offers to help a handful of other local Lost Boys who are also missing teeth.

Over time, new discoveries are no longer sources of fear or embarrassment for the Lost Boys, but mostly sources of humor. Two months after their arrival, some of the guys and I share a pizza and I ask them what foods they now like or dislike. In the middle of devouring his second slice, Gabriel pauses from eating to answer my question.

"I do not like cheese!" he states emphatically.

"Gabriel! What do you think all that white stuff on your pizza is?" I say, laughing.

"This is cheese?" he asks.

During another get-together, James complains about gaining weight. In the Sudanese culture it's the wife's job to fatten her husband, and no woman will want James if he becomes overweight before marriage, Daniel explains to me.

"What have you been eating?" I ask James. He tells me that every day there is cake and ice cream for someone's birthday at the retirement home where he now works.

"But I thought you guys didn't like sweet foods," I say, thinking back on the Safeway bakery worker's failed attempt at offering a culinary treat.

"Ohhh no, Mom. I now like cake and ice cream very much. I eat it every day!" he says without a trace of irony in his voice.

"Well, no wonder you've gained weight!" I say.

"Cake makes you fat?" James replies. He seems genuinely surprised by this discovery.

It is a real joy to watch the Lost Boys grow into their American lives. Jeff and I introduce them to video-game arcades and the movies, and in return they teach us how to properly kill a rhinoceros. (Dig a large ditch, fill it with spears pointing straight up, goad the rhinoceros into chasing you toward said ditch, then jump out of the way at the last minute. Once the rhinoceros has impaled itself on the spears in the ditch, attack from above with more spears. Cook till tender. Season to taste.)

At times, I find the discrepancies in our two lifestyles so vast that I must squelch the desire to simply move these boys into our home and take care of them on a daily basis. While I know it's an unreasonable plan, I often imagine what it'd be like to legally adopt one—Daniel, perhaps?—and give him the same opportunities, the same level of comfort afforded his American counterparts. But then I learn from one of the resettlement counselors that self-reliance is a critical aspect in helping refugees transition to their new lives, and years of immigration experience suggest that independent living is best. And so I continue to make Costco runs, and drive them to job interviews, and take them shopping for appropriate work clothing, and slip them each a few twenty-dollar bills here and there.

Because that's what we mothers do.

37

NOVEMBER 4, 2001. JEFF AND I STAND at the starting line, which isn't really a line so much as a massive herd of people. Many of the runners are pulling one leg at a time toward their behinds, or stretching to the side, one hand extending overhead, the other on a hip. Some hop up and down or wear garbage bags to keep warm. Others are already peeling off the extra clothing they're wearing, tossing sweatpants and warm-up jackets onto the lawn area to be collected, laundered, and donated to nonprofit groups that assist the homeless. The temperatures have risen a bit since we first arrived on Staten Island a few hours ago. The air is crisp, but the skies are clear. A perfect day to run 26.2 miles with 30,000 strangers, all of whom feel like family right now. A year and a half ago, I couldn't have fathomed being here, preparing to run my seventh marathon.

The 10:50 a.m. start time nears, and I feel a quickening within me: at once nervous and excited, smiling and tearing up. I stand mute, in awe, as the runners around me sing "The Star Spangled Banner" and white doves are released overhead. In no other marathon have I felt such a surge of prerace emotion. It feels like graduation, an ending and a beginning.

"This is it," Jeff says. It's not lost on me that he said the same words as I was being pushed in a wheelchair from the doctor's office to the hospital for an emergency C-section, and again six weeks later as I was being pushed in a wheelchair from the hospital to go home. Today, there is no wheelchair. Today, my legs will carry me.

The announcer counts down from ten to one over the loudspeaker, and we count with him. At one, a gun goes off and the energy of the crowd increases. We all push forward as a single body, but after a few seconds we slow, then stop. I realize the only runners leaping forward for now are those a quarter-mile ahead of us, the elite runners seeded at the front.

Jeff points to the top of the Verrazano-Narrows Bridge, where sharpshooters stand poised with rifles. The horror of 9/11 less than eight weeks old, it occurs to me that this race—with runners representing nearly a hundred different countries—is a perfect terrorist target, a perfectly atrocious opportunity to spit on the international goodwill that has blanketed the United States since the first plane rammed the World Trade Center.

"Wow," I say. "That's new."

We continue taking baby steps forward, my gaze intermittently returning to the National Guardsmen overhead, and five minutes later, we reach the official starting line. Making our way onto the bridge, I laugh when I see male runners lining the sides of the bridge and urinating into the waters below.

"Wanna join them?" I ask Jeff. "It's a tradition." I remember seeing hordes of peeing men on the same bridge the first time I ran this race thirteen years ago. At first I was surprised, and a little disgusted, that so many men had forgotten to use the port-o-potties in the prerace area, but I soon learned it was a long-standing New York City Marathon tradition to use the bridge instead.

"I think I'll pass," Jeff says. He has never been one to cave to the pressures of convention.

The mass of runners begins to disperse, so Jeff and I increase our pace to a jog, but halfway across the bridge we stop dead in our tracks. A wave of sadness washes over me and I work my way through the crowd to the left as if drawn by a magnetic force, then stare, speechless, at the noticeable gap on the southern end of the Manhattan skyline. It looks like a tooth extraction, the gums not yet grown over the wound. I pull the disposable camera I bought yesterday from my hydration backpack and snap a few pictures, feeling intrusive as I do so.

After two miles we exit the bridge onto Brooklyn soil, the second of the five boroughs we'll run through today. In sharp contrast to the subdued patter of running shoes that we heard on the bridge, we now hear a crescendo of cheers from people—black, Hispanic, Caucasian—all urging us on. We pull off our warm-up jackets and toss them on the side of the road. They too will be collected, laundered, and donated to those who could use a bit more warmth.

In every marathon I've run in the past, I've always worn a shirt that read *Go Lauren Go!* and it never failed to prompt spectators to cheer for me by name, an effective form of motivation during the seemingly endless miles. For this race, I changed my shirt's message to reflect the underlying sentiment of my near-fatal experience: *Hey Lauren, you're alive!* Jeff's shirt acknowledges our shared sense of gratitude toward the hundreds of anonymous people who made my survival possible: *Thank you, blood donors!*

"Go, Lauren!" I hear from the crowd.

"You can do it, Lauren!" someone else yells.

"Thank you!" I call to no one in particular. I realize I can't stop smiling.

"Hey, Lauren!" someone shouts. "You're alive!"

That does it. I begin crying, though the smile never leaves my face. Jeff turns to me and squeezes my shoulder as we jog side by side. "You okay?"

I shake my head yes and wipe away the tears.

"Thank you, blood donors?" someone yells, her voice trailing off into a question, making me laugh.

With the field of runners now sufficiently spread out, Jeff and I jog at a consistent, though slow, pace—an eleven-minute mile. He follows my lead on how fast we run, where on the road we position ourselves, and when we stop to stretch out our calves against the curb. This is my race and, as he's told me repeatedly, he's here to support me.

Jeff hates running. When I invited him to run the Los Angeles Marathon with me three months after we'd met, he agreed, even showed excitement over the prospect of accomplishing such a feat. We trained together for six months, and on race day Jeff was strong and crossed the finish line with ease. He could've finished much sooner had he not insisted on keeping pace with me when I began to feel the effects of dehydration at mile nineteen. Afterward, over several beers and a celebratory dinner of cheeseburgers and fries, I was reveling in the high of our shared accomplishment.

"Wasn't that great!" I declared more than asked.

"Sure," he said. "And I never want to do it again."

We laughed, and I agreed never to ask him to run another marathon with me.

Four years later, he began to join me on my training runs for New York. "You don't need to do this," I told him. And I meant it, mostly.

"What kind of complete wuss would I be," he said, "if my almost-died wife runs twenty-six miles while her husband stands on the sidelines yelling *Go honey?*"

He had a point.

I run in the center of the road to the side of the painted divider lines, which have a slight but noticeable elevation to them. The side of the road is equally treacherous because the pavement slopes toward the gutter area. A smooth flat surface is best for my somewhat precarious joints. But now we're running through a densely populated working-class neighborhood and children line the curb, their hands extended in hopes of high-fiving as many passing runners as possible. I work my way toward the right side of the road, Jeff following. I extend my arm, smiling and crying as children smack my hand and the adults surrounding them clap and cheer.

Chants of *Go Lauren!* and *Hey, Lauren, you're alive!* ring in my ears as my vision gets blurrier. I pretend I'm running down the corridor of a hospital toward the exit, that all these people are my doctors and nurses cheering me on as I leave my death-bed behind. I'm now sobbing uncontrollably, my breathing interrupted by halting gasps. Jeff seems to understand the sensory overload of my being here today, of running this race, as he reaches his arm behind me and pats my back.

At the next intersection, a fire truck is parked at the side of the road, firemen standing on top of it, clapping for the runners. And we runners, as if on cue, look up at the firemen and clap for them. Both runners and firemen wipe away tears.

"On your left!" I hear from behind. "Running for charity! On your left!"

I glance over my shoulder to see a runner sprint past me along the side of the road. His pace suggests that he should've been seeded with the faster runners up ahead. I think nothing of it until I read the paper the following morning and learn that he's a firefighter who ran the marathon to honor the 343 firefighters who died in the Twin Towers. JP Morgan Chase bank agreed to donate $5 for every runner he passed during the race. He started dead last, but by the time he crossed the finish fine, Larry Parker of Ladder 129 in Queens raised over $118,000 for the Uniformed Firefighters Association Widows' and Children's Fund.

Somewhere around mile eleven, I question my ability to finish the race. The soles of my feet feel as if they're burning. On this stretch of the racecourse, the number of spectators has diminished. Gone is the ethnically diverse crowd that packed the roadside. We've entered a Hasidic neighborhood, one that doesn't seem to share the rest of Brooklyn's enthusiasm for marathon day. Bearded men in long black coats and black hats walk with purpose along the sidewalks, occasionally glancing at the passing runners. Boys with long curled *payot* dangling from under their yarmulkes run along the side of the road, showing slightly more interest in the race than their elders. I slow my pace to a walk, a luxury I've never allowed myself in previous marathons, fearing that if I go any slower or sit on the curb for a brief rest, I'll never get started again. I remind myself that the pain I now feel is nothing compared to having a liver biopsy performed through my neck. It helps.

Half a mile later, I begin jogging, and soon we enter the borough of Queens. Once more, we pass through immigrant neighborhoods, and festive crowds cheer from the sidelines. At street corners, bands of musicians play alongside fire trucks packed with cheering firefighters. My eyes fill with tears every time we pass another one.

Reaching the Queensboro Bridge, we run onto red outdoor carpeting that's been placed over the metal grating on the sides of the bridge to prevent injuries. My searing feet feel some re-lief, but now my calves ache from the slight upward slope of the bridge. I bargain with my feet and legs. If they'll carry me to the top of the arc, I'll rest them before starting on the downward slope. They agree, and a quarter-mile later I tell Jeff it's time for a break. I lie on the center divider of the bridge and lift my feet straight up toward the sky, the relief palpable and immediate. I close my eyes and feel the unobstructed sunshine of a crisp clear New York City day on my body. Jeff snaps a photo of me, my arms wrapped behind my knees, feet overhead, and a huge smile on my face. Later, when I view this photo, I'll marvel at how comfortable I appear to be.

After a two-minute break, I slowly rise to standing. Stretch-ing my calves against the center divider, I do a few side bends.

We begin jogging down the bridge toward Manhattan, and except for the sound of feet hitting the pavement, there is very little noise. No fans are allowed on the bridges, and this one is nearly a mile long. The faces of the runners around us seem to reflect the same sense of a death march that I feel. With ten more miles to go, Jeff's face tells me he's feeling ragged too.

"One of my favorite parts is coming up," I say to offer a bit of encouragement. "Once we get off this bridge, there'll be tons of spectators." He nods, and we run on in silence.

At the bottom of the bridge we make a sharp left, then another. I hear the crowds, though I can't yet see them. One more left turn and the field of runners empties onto First Avenue, headed north. The sidewalks are jammed with people cheering, many holding American flags or signs made of poster board so their friends in the race can pick them out of the crowd. The bars and restaurants that line the street are packed, their doors and windows opening onto the marathon route. I see diners eating brunch and sipping mimosas at patio tables, and I imagine how nice it would be to trade places with one of them.

Someone holds half-bananas for passing runners, and Jeff and I each take one. I mouth the words *Thank you* because speaking will take too much effort. We eat our bananas while jogging, then toss the peels toward the gutter. I hear my name being called out from both sides of the street, and again I'm glad I personalized my shirt. A woman jogging nearby leans in front of me, glancing at my chest, and laughs.

"So that's it!" she says. "I've been hearing people call my name left and right and I finally realized it must be someone's shirt!" She thanks me and continues to run at my side.

"Happy to help," I say.

"This is my first marathon. If I ever do another one, I'm definitely putting my name on my shirt."

We continue on, Jeff on my left and my new friend on my right, the other Lauren and I sharing a laugh every time we hear our name called from the crowd.

"Lauren!" I hear from the right side of the road. I smile and keep running.

"LAUREN LARSEN!" shouts the same voice.

I scan the crowd and see Joey at the curbside, smiling and waving wildly. Jeff and I move toward him, across thousands of flattened paper cups from the last water station. I turn back toward the other Lauren, who has kept pace with us for well over a mile.

"Sorry," I say. "Gotta go!"

"Thanks again!" she yells back.

I haven't seen Joey since his brief visit to Boulder a year ago, when my twisted intestines put me in the hospital. He and his girlfriend step off the curb, and I embrace each of them in an awkward hug, trying to keep from soaking them with my sweat.

"When I didn't see you at mile sixteen, I thought we'd missed you," I say.

"This was the closest we could get," Joey says.

The four of us stand together for another minute, goofy smiles adorning our faces, as if we haven't seen one another in years and our meeting was coincidental. They seem to be as excited about the race as we are, fully understanding how monumental this occasion is for me.

"We ought to get going so we don't stiffen up," Jeff says, and we all hug one last time.

"See you at dinner!" I yell over my shoulder as we work our way into the center of the road again. Less than a mile later, it happens again.

"Lauren!" I hear. I smile but don't waste energy turning my head toward the spectators.

"LAUREN AND JEFF!" shouts the same voice. This time it's our friend Monica. She stands on the left side of the road holding a huge cardboard sign with our names on it. We stop and hug, and a nearby spectator takes our photo with my camera.

"See you tonight!" I say, slowly merging into the throng of runners again.

Buoyed by the crowds and my friends, I feel a second wind invigorating my body. I increase my pace and let the energy of the city carry me along the next several miles. These are my people, the same type of twenty- and thirty-something professionals I spent weekends with when I lived in a suburb of New York over a decade ago. Now, the hubris that permeated the yuppie scene all those years ago is subdued, the scent of the smoldering towers still wafting in the air a few miles to the south. When I first ran the New York City Marathon at age twenty-six, it was a sense of pride and the anticipation of bragging rights at the office the next day that sustained me along the course. Today, it's a sense of humanity, a sense of love I feel for these New Yorkers, that propels me forward.

Somewhere around 98th Street, I get a crippling charley horse in my left leg. I limp to the side of the road and sit on the curb in front of a hospital. Jeff sits next to me and massages my calf, stretches my foot toward my knee. We've been running for four and a half hours and are still seven miles from the finish. The soles of my feet burn, my legs feel like overcooked noodles, my upper body aches, and my face stings from evaporated sweat. I slip off my CamelBak water pack and lie back on the ground. Jeff removes my sneakers and rubs my sweaty feet. In no other race have I felt this depleted with so much distance yet to run. My body wants out. I could easily limp a block to the west and catch a cab to our hotel on 7th Avenue. No one would fault me for it. Some would tell me it was the smart thing to do, reminding me how ambitious it was to think of running a marathon so soon after my illness.

"Should we quit?" Jeff asks, his tone suggestive, as if he wanted to say *We should quit*. He knows me well, knows how stubborn I can be, how determined, especially in the face of doubt. He knows better than to tell me what to do during this particular race, my comeback. I leave the question hanging between us as I lie on the sidewalk, feeling the coolness of the cement on my back, noticing the sun dipping low through the tree branches above.

Five minutes pass in silence, as I reflect on what this race means to me, how my personal give-back campaign propelled me forward with every word of encouragement scratched in the margins of reply forms I received from friends and strangers alike. Since launching my effort eight months ago, I've raised nearly $35,000 and 535 pints of blood. I know none of my supporters would demand the return of their donation if I failed to cross the finish line, but I want more than anything to make good on my end of the bargain. I've never dropped out of a race. And I'm not about to start today.

"Let's go," I say. I sit up and put on my running shoes. Jeff stands, then turns to pull me to my feet. When my quadriceps fail to assist in rousing me, Jeff moves behind me and hoists me up from my armpits. We both laugh at the absurdity of the situation I've put us in, the expectations I've placed upon myself and then broadcast to the world through my letter campaign. Jeff slips my CamelBak onto my back as he would a coat, gives me a quick kiss, and we walk-jog our way into the now sparse field of runners.

Soon we cross over the East River for the second time today and enter The Bronx. I tell Jeff that this is where Carol almost dropped out of the race back in 1988. Her knee hurt, and she wasn't sure if she could make it. I started to jog ahead of her, wondering if she'd stop and take the subway back into Manhattan. A few minutes later, I heard her calling to me, and soon she was keeping pace. For the remaining six miles, I repeated little statements of encouragement, as much for myself as for her. We crossed the finish line together, and Carol promptly retired from distance running.

Now, it's Jeff's turn to play the role of motivational coach, while *I* wonder if I'm going to make it to the end. But once more, the crowds pull me along. The Bronx is wild with excitement, even though all the elite runners have long since passed through and are probably showered and enjoying a cold beer at their hotels. Our time in this borough is brief, and a mile later we're back in Manhattan, working our way south from the Madison Avenue Bridge. It's dusk, and the crowds in East Harlem are almost nonexistent. A few men sit on the stoops of small liquor stores, cradling paper bags that I suspect hold quarts of beer. Most of the businesses are closed, locked accordion gates stretching the width of their storefronts and graffiti adorning nearby brick walls. Several children stand in a group on the left side of the road, yelling to passing runners and handing something to those who venture close. I work my way toward them and accept a piece of chewing gum. Though dehydrated, I feel tears on my face.

The northern tip of Central Park comes into view, which means we're getting closer. Running south on 5th Avenue in the dark, I repeat *Almost there, almost there* like a mantra. We pass the twenty-three-mile marker.

Almost there, almost there.

My gait has a slight hobble to it, my pace a fourteen-minute mile at best. But now I'm confident that I will cross that finish line. We pass the twenty-four-mile marker.

Almost there, almost there.

I wonder aloud what our current projected race time is and whether we'll make it to the end in under six hours. There was a time when I believed that a five-hour marathon wasn't worth lacing up one's running shoes for. Right now, a sub-six-hour marathon sounds pretty good, and I'm hopeful that we'll achieve it. Massive time clocks are stationed at every 10K point along the route, as well as at the halfway point. The next one should be coming up soon, at twenty-four and eight-tenths miles. Just as the clock comes into view, we see its yellow illuminated numbers go dark. Then several men in jumpsuits lay the clock on its back and begin disassembling its legs and loading them into a white pickup truck.

"You're fucking kidding me!" Jeff says, and we both start laughing. "They're hauling away the time clocks?"

"We're pathetic," I say, though both of us know that I feel nothing but triumphant.

As we pass the twenty-five-mile marker, the crowd along the roadside thickens, kept clear of the racecourse by police barricades. Women in fur coats and doormen in fancy uniforms adorn the wide sidewalks behind the spectators. The air is electric as we turn right onto Central Park South.

"You're almost there!" we hear over and over again from strangers, who clap and cheer us on.

"That's what they said four miles ago!" I yell back. The crowd laughs in appreciation. I no longer need my *almost there* incantation because we truly are almost there. We make another right turn into the park.

"We're coming up on the best part," I say to Jeff.

I've told him a number of times about the finish line of the New York City Marathon and how much fun it was when Carol and I crossed it years ago. Bleachers had been erected along the last stretch of the course and they were filled with cheering fans, with loud music blasting in the background. An announcer acknowledged individual runners over a PA system by reading whatever was on their shirts: bib numbers, messages, or names. I remember what a thrill it was to hear his booming voice announcing our arrival. *And here come Carol and Lauren, folks! Go, Carol, go! Go, Lauren, go!* We held hands and reached high in the air as we crossed the finish line, smiling up at the thirty or so official race photographers on the scaffolding overhead. A flock of race volunteers urged us to keep moving forward to prevent a traffic jam among the many runners crowding the finish area. They guided us into the proper queues for our finisher's medals, our disposable Mylar blankets to prevent hypothermia, and then our goodie bags containing an apple, granola bar, and sandwich.

But thirteen years ago, I finished the marathon in just over four hours. Today, we're coming in at six hours and eight minutes. It's five o'clock and the November sky is pitch black. No music is playing because the PA system has been turned off. No fans line the final stretch of the racecourse because the bleachers have been disassembled and stacked, waiting to be carted away. A few fans linger at the finish line, and only a couple of race photographers are in sight. A wheelchair entrant skirts past us with three yards to go, and I imagine him chuckling under his breath about lapping yet another able-bodied racer. Only a handful of volunteers remains at the finish area, which is flooded with bright lights from the scaffolding above. Jeff and I cross the finish line and stop in our tracks, bending forward and resting our hands on our knees to catch our breath. Of the 23,664 runners who will complete the race today, my finishing place is 22,758—my worst marathon performance to date. And the one I'm most proud of. We stand tall and embrace, my tears flowing freely as I clutch the back of Jeff's shirt to keep my arms from dropping.

"We did it," I say. "We did it."

One of the race volunteers, an older woman, approaches us and stands quietly off to the side until we're ready to allow her into our private moment. Then gently, almost reverently, she places a finisher's medal around each of our necks. She sees the disposable camera sticking out of my CamelBak and asks if we'd like her to take our picture. I tell her yes, and Jeff and I stand side by side, our arms around one another, and smile. This will become, and will remain, my all-time favorite photo of the two of us.

She hands my camera back to me, and once more Jeff folds me into his arms. I'm overcome with the emotional significance of this event, the enormity of what Jeff and I have accomplished, not just today, but since the day my daughter was removed, limp and silent, from my womb. This is much more than runner's high. It's survivor's gratitude.

38

I HADN'T PLANNED ON BECOMING a national advocate for the cause, hadn't planned on being featured in public service announcements or testifying before the Food and Drug Administration or traveling the country to give keynote addresses about the incredible impact people can have by donating an hour of their time and a pint of their blood. I thought my efforts related to blood donation would cease when I crossed the finish line of the marathon, when my personal give-back effort concluded. I didn't plan on any of this, but as I've learned, sometimes things just happen. And a couple months after the marathon, something big was about to happen.

Jeff and I board a plane to Dallas, where I'm to be presented with a national award from America's Blood Centers for my marathon campaign. Jim MacPherson meets me in the hotel lobby before the event and tells me that a bigwig from Johnson & Johnson will be in the audience that evening.

"I recently asked him for a million-dollar donation for our foundation," Jim says of the Johnson & Johnson representative. "So do me a favor and make him cry when you give your acceptance speech tonight. It might seal the deal."

During the banquet, a full program makes conversation close to impossible. Toward the end of the dessert course, my name is announced. I make my way to the stage, give a brief talk, and return to my seat. Soon after, the banquet concludes and I'm surrounded by people—mostly blood center presidents—shaking my hand, hugging me, and offering congratulations. As Jeff and I walk back to our hotel room, he hands me a place card with *Willard Nielsen* printed on it and a handwritten e-mail address beneath the name.

"*Willard?*" I say. "Like the rat movie?"

"Yep," Jeff says. "He was seated next to you at dinner."

"The older guy?"

"Yep."

"I didn't get to talk to him much, but he seemed nice."

"Get in touch with him. He wants to help you."

"Help me what?"

"I don't know, but he works for Johnson & Johnson. He didn't have any business cards with him, so he gave me that."

I have no idea that Willard—Bill, once I get to know him—is the worldwide head of public affairs for the global healthcare giant. But he is. I have no idea that Johnson & Johnson has a deep commitment to supporting volunteer blood donation. But they do. And I certainly have no idea that Bill will fly me to the company's world headquarters, have me meet with the chairman of the board, and offer to financially support my advocacy efforts—in addition to the million dollars he's already committed to America's Blood Centers—so that the pro bono talks I've been doing sporadically can expand to a full-time national speaking tour. But he does, and it will. As a jaded former marketer, I wonder *What's the catch?*

"Where are you going to tattoo the J&J logo?" I jokingly ask Bill during our first meeting after he offers to underwrite my work. "Across my forehead?"

He laughs. "You don't need to mention us at all," he says. "Just go out there and do more of what you've been doing. It's good stuff."

Months later, I'm speaking at a blood-banking conference on the East Coast, and one of the other panelists in my session talks about introducing blood recipients to some of their actual blood donors as a way to raise public awareness about the cause. I hadn't realized that was possible, since blood donation is a highly regulated and anonymous process. At the break, I duck out of the conference hall and call Lisa Bloch at Blood Centers of the Pacific. With an insouciant demeanor and a wicked sense of humor, Lisa is the Sarah Silverman of blood banking. The moment she answers, I all but scream, "I want to meet my blood donors!"

"I don't think that's legal," she says, laughing.

"It is! I just learned all about it. Virginia Blood Services is doing it, and they got the idea from Bonfils Blood Center, who's done it for several years now." I know Lisa well enough by now to understand that nagging alone won't gain her support. The key word in getting to yes is *fun*. "C'mon," I say. "It'll be fun!"

"Okay, okay," she says, relenting. "But only because it's you."

During the planning of the blood center's inaugural Patient-Donor Reunion, as Lisa dubs it, she calls regularly to tell me how things are progressing.

"Damn it, Larsen, this event of yours is killing me," she says one day. "I've been calling your blood donors to invite them, and I end up crying my eyes out. At work! Do you know what this is doing to my reputation as a coldhearted bitch?"

Another day, she calls full of excitement. All but three of the donors she was able to track down said they'd love to meet someone whose life their blood had saved. The event is shaping up nicely. I'll get to thank some of my donors face to face, and the blood center will get some press coverage to help alleviate the blood shortages they face daily. As for the donors, my wish is that by meeting Jeff, Clare, and me, they'll receive confirmation that the seemingly minor act of donating blood makes an impact far greater than they can imagine. In my case, they not only saved a new mom, they saved an entire family.

On January 14, 2004, I wait, nervous, in the hallway of the hospital where I was treated after Clare's birth. Grabbing a stack of napkins off a nearby catering table, I dab the sweat from my upper lip and forehead.

"Deep breaths, honey," Jeff says, rubbing my shoulders.

"I can't believe this is happening, that I'm actually about to meet them."

"You'll be fine. Just relax."

"How's my lipstick?"

"Looks good."

Lisa opens the door and pokes her head into the hallway. "Just a few more minutes," she says. "Dr. Osorio is almost finished with his remarks."

With the door cracked, I can hear Bob sharing his perspective about the many blood transfusions I received during my illness. His point is simple: Without them, no matter how good my medical team was, I'd be dead.

Clare is already in the room with my mother, stepfather, brother, and girlfriends Pam and Sabra. Some of my former nurses and doctors are there too, along with more people from the blood center, several newspaper reporters, and camera crews from the local TV stations. I already know that sitting in the first two rows, directly in front of the lectern where I'm about to speak, are twenty-one strangers—no, *angels*—who saved my life with their blood donations four years ago.

"I think I'm going to cry," I say to Jeff, my giddiness shifting to panic.

"You can do this, hon."

"Glad I wore waterproof mascara."

"This is supposed to be fun. Just think of it as another one of your talks."

"Okay, we're ready for you," Lisa says, again leaning her head into the hallway. She has purposely kept me out of the room until now to build anticipation. Stepping through the door, I feel like the winning contestant on *The Dating Game*: overjoyed, overwhelmed, and hopeful that they'll like me now that they're finally meeting me in person.

I hear the click of cameras as I walk to the front of the room. Jeff sits in a chair off to the side and motions for Clare to join him. Lisa introduces me and steps away from the microphone. Usually proud of my ability to speak off the cuff, today I pull two pages of typed notes from my jacket pocket and smooth them out on the lectern, purposely giving myself time to regain my composure. I'm unable to look directly at the first two rows of people for fear of breaking down before I deliver my remarks.

When I finally begin speaking I can hear the quiver in my voice, can feel a slight trembling in my arms as I grip my notes. I stop, take a deep breath, and allow myself to look at one, then another and another of my blood donors, whose eyes are as watery as mine. A Hispanic gentleman, my age or perhaps a few years younger, sits in the middle of the second row, in his lap a bouquet of flowers. Near him is a young Caucasian woman, early twenties at most, wearing a blue striped sweater, her straight blonde hair tucked behind her ears. I'm struck by how wonderfully ordinary this group of extraordinary people appears, and I'm no longer feeling nervous. What I'm feeling is love, pure and simple. I'm not a game show contestant. I'm a mom, one who is grateful beyond words for these people who gave me the chance to know the precocious four-year-old who sits on her daddy's lap nibbling the candy necklace we bought her yesterday. I continue sharing my story, and by the time I reach my closing remarks, I don't care that I'm openly wiping away tears.

"Please know that not a day has gone by that I don't appreciate what you've given me." I say. "The world needs more people like you. You not only care about others, you actually take the time to express that concern in a very tangible and meaningful way."

Jeff leads Clare to the podium, and my daughter, half her candy necklace devoured, delivers the closing message.

"Thank you, *bwood* donors, for saving my mommy."

Lisa joins us and announces that she'd like to bring each of my donors to the front of the room, one by one. "There's an interesting story behind the first donor I'm going to call up," she says. "He's so loyal to the cause that Lauren received not one, but two pints of blood from him: one that was already available when she first got sick, and another when his next appointment to give blood arrived. Raul Alfaro, would you please come up?"

The Hispanic man with the bouquet of flowers makes his way toward me and wraps me in a bear hug. After handing me the flowers, he hugs Jeff, then Clare. We're all crying, but that doesn't stop me from reaching behind the podium, where earlier I'd stashed some supplies. I pull out a novelty-store angel halo and place it on Raul's head. Now we're all crying *and* laughing. Clare approaches Raul and offers him a framed Certificate of Thanks that's signed by her, first name only and with a beginner's awkward penmanship. For that, she receives a second hug.

Raul remains up front with us as Lisa calls each of my donors up for a hug, a halo, and a Certificate of Thanks. Among them are a postman, a scientist, an attorney, a software engineer. James, one of my donors who drove four hours to get to the ceremony, hands me a small box and asks me to open it. Inside is a pendant made from a flat green stone with red spots, a bloodstone, he explains. I thank him and perch a halo on his head. He joins our ever-expanding group as Lisa calls the next person's name.

Blanche tells me she's there on behalf of her husband, Roger, who's out of town. I learn that, like me, Blanche nearly bled to death during childbirth fourteen years earlier, which prompted her husband to begin donating regularly. Though not one of my donors, she gets a halo nonetheless.

Another of my donors asks me if I've been swearing more since receiving his blood. "I'm from New Jersey!" I say. "I don't need any more help in that department!" We share a laugh as I plop a halo on his head.

Athena, the young woman in the striped sweater, is one of the last people called up. I learn that she was only seventeen when she donated the blood that helped save my life.

"I knew there must've been a reason I've been listening to Britney Spears music ever since my illness," I say. Athena blushes, probably embarrassed on my behalf for the inept pop cultural reference.

When all the donors have joined me up front, we link arms for a photo, everyone trying to hold his or her smile long enough for the photographers to capture a decent group shot. In her event invitations, Lisa had made reference to "a family reunion like no other," and her choice of analogies couldn't have been more apt. This big assortment of people, spanning a number of ethnicities and generations, feels like a part of me. We hug and talk and exchange addresses, and when the last of my angels has departed, I sit for the first time in hours and devour a box lunch from the hospital's catering service.

Jeff, Clare, and I have been awake since five in the morning to appear on a live television show before the Patient-Donor Reunion, so by the time we return to our hotel room we're exhausted. We order an early dinner through room service and fall into bed by eight.

The next morning, there's another early wake-up call, this time at three-thirty. While Jeff and Clare sleep, I tiptoe around the hotel room getting dressed, then take a cab across town to a television studio. For the next several hours, I'm beamed into news programs and morning shows across the country, one after another after another, giving back-to-back interviews about National Volunteer Blood Donor Month and what it was like to personally thank the strangers who saved my life. I have trouble keeping the names of the news anchors straight and I can't remember which of my talking points I've already shared in each interview. It's fast-paced and exhausting, and I'm having a blast. When the last of the scheduled interviews is complete, I sigh with relief and unhook the microphone from my jacket lapel.

This is not the life I'd envisioned for myself during all those years of climbing the corporate ladder and setting goals and having one-year, five-year, and ten-year plans. Yet here I am on this unexpected path as an advocate for volunteer blood donation, taking it day by day and simply being open to whatever interesting opportunities arise. I can still remember in vivid detail the shock that rippled through me when I awoke in the hospital and was told I'd been receiving regular blood transfusions for weeks, how I convinced myself that I'd die of AIDS as a result, and how frightened and angry I was about that.

I now see that the ignorance that gripped me back then was based on a lack of understanding about the blood supply and medical advancements in safety testing, combined with a touch of lingering encephalopathy. And yet in my travels and talks, I see that misperceptions about receiving and donating blood are still perpetuated through the myths that exist: that giving blood isn't safe. That receiving blood isn't safe. That it hurts. That someone else will do it. That it's not a cause I need care about because it won't happen to me. This last misperception is, I believe, the most dangerous because it breeds exactly the type of indifference to the cause that I myself possessed, the type that makes "inconvenience" an acceptable excuse for not helping. My blood donation record prior to becoming a recipient is embarrassing, if not shameful, and now that I understand its importance, it's too late. I'm no longer a viable donor.

"Check it out!" says Jeff when I return to the hotel room later that morning. He holds up the front page of the *San Fran-*

cisco Chronicle's local news section. *Blood Type A-ngels* reads the headline. *Recipient meets donors who helped save her life.* A photo of me with my "angels" takes up a good portion of the page, with another photo of Raul and me hugging below that one. Jeff turns the page to show me two more photos from the event and several more columns of copy.

"Wow! Great coverage," I say. I notice a stack of maybe twenty or more copies of the same paper on the coffee table. "Where'd those come from?" I ask.

"You don't want to know," Jeff says.

"You didn't," I say, imagining my husband sneaking from one hotel room door to the next, stealing newspapers that belong to the other guests.

"I did," he says, a guilty smile on his face. "And I would've gotten more, but I didn't want to roam too far with Clare asleep in the room." I glance in the bedroom and see that my daughter is still sleeping soundly.

By noon, I'm back in bed for a few more hours of rest while Jeff and Clare go shopping with Sabra. They return, sneaking a case of Veuve Clicquot and giant platters of sushi into our hotel suite using my oversized pull-along suitcase. Clare carries a bouquet of balloons. Multiple trips to and from Sabra's car yield more food: cheeses and crackers, olives, a fruit tray, rolls and sliced roast beef—all contraband, given the hotel's policy requiring guests to use their internal catering group for parties. Clare and Jeff adorn the suite with paper Chinese lanterns, curly foil garland, silk butterflies, and other mismatched decorations my daughter picked out at the party supply warehouse. Sabra arranges food on serving platters she brought from her home, while I order two bottles of cheap champagne from room service, asking them to include several dozen champagne glasses. When they arrive, I feign innocence, then include a huge gratuity on the check, hoping my generosity will buy silence about the party that is obviously about to take place.

Half an hour later, there's another knock at the door, and I open it to find the same room service runner with chocolate-covered strawberries and another bottle of champagne. "A gift," he says, rolling the table into our suite. Jeff picks up the card by the platter of strawberries. "It's from Liz and Rick. *Wish we could be there for the celebration*," he says. "Too bad they moved. I miss them."

Ten minutes pass, and another room service delivery arrives with another platter of chocolate-covered strawberries. Jeff reads the card. "From Jim MacPherson and all your friends at America's Blood Centers," he says. "Nice!"

Soon the phone rings and we give our friends on the line our room number. Clare greets them at the door, wearing her yellow Disney princess gown and a plastic tiara, bright red lipstick smeared around her mouth in what looks like a parody of Courtney Love. We repeat this process over and over until the suite is packed with old neighbors and work colleagues and grad school pals, many of whom we haven't seen since we moved from San Francisco four years ago. Lisa arrives late, waving a VHS tape overhead when she spots me across the room. Popping the tape into the video player, she summons everyone to the television.

"We got coverage of Lauren's story on all the major local stations," she announces to the group. "The phones at the blood center have been ringing off the hook." This is great news, she explains, because the current shortage of blood in the Bay Area is so severe, hospitals have had to postpone operations, including an open-heart surgery a few days ago.

Lisa pushes a button on the video player, and Jeff and I add ancillary commentary as four different news stories about the Patient-Donor Reunion play on the screen. *That guy was awesome. She was only seventeen! Oh god, did I really say 'heap of trouble?' There's Bob!* When the camera zooms in on Clare as she thanks all the blood donors, our friends say *awww* in unison, and my daughter, perched on Jeff's hip, beams with pride. When the tape ends, Lisa lifts her champagne glass and turns toward me.

"I know this may sound awful, but I'll say it anyway," she says. "I'm really sorry you had to get sick and go through everything you did. But *since* you did, I'm really glad it happened in my city!" The room erupts in laughter, signaling that Lisa has just been accepted into our circle of friends.

"Happy birthday, Lauren!" she adds, and we all raise our glasses. My forty-second today, this is, without question, the best birthday of my life.

39

I USED TO BELIEVE my illness was a rare one. But in the years since, I've learned more about the prevalence of preeclampsia, that upward of eight percent of all pregnancies are complicated by it. Now, I find myself frustrated by the lack of progress toward a definitive cure for this age-old killer, so when I'm invited to speak about preeclampsia at a medical conference in the fall of 2004, I gladly accept.

On the flight home from the conference, I have a layover in Chicago. While I wait to pay for a plate of Chinese fast food at the airport, a woman in line looks at me and says, "I know someone you need to meet." Confused, I look at my tray of food—fried rice, spring rolls, and a Pepsi—and wonder if she's about to recommend a nutritionist.

"Sorry," she says, laughing. "I was at your talk yesterday. I tried to find you afterward, but you'd already left. Have you ever met Anne Garrett? She started the Preeclampsia Foundation."

"There's a *foundation?*" I say.

"They've been up and running a few years now. You really ought to meet her. And Eleni Tsigas, the head of the board."

We pay for our respective meals and then swap business cards, she promising to e-mail me with contact information for these two women.

Weeks later, I'm on the phone with Eleni, formerly a public relations executive, who shares the horrific story of her first pregnancy: the rush to the hospital when she sensed something was wrong, the nine hours she waited for a diagnosis—two of which were due to the radiologist being "too busy" to give prompt attention to her ultrasound results—and then finally being transferred to a major hospital across town, where she was told her baby had died in utero during the ambulance ride. I listen, stunned. This sort of stuff isn't supposed to happen, not in this country, not in this century.

I spend hours on the Preeclampsia Foundation's Web site, reading story after story about women like me, women who thought they were having normal pregnancies—*normal* discomfort, *normal* swelling, *normal* weight gain—only to learn there was nothing normal about their symptoms. Many lost their babies, some lost their lives, and all of them lost any naïveté they might have had about the ease of pregnancy. Along with the details of their experiences with preeclampsia and HELLP Syndrome, many of the people who posted their stories—women terrified of getting pregnant again, men who became widowers at the same time they became fathers—questioned what they could've or should've or might've done differently. Discernible in many of the narratives was a sense of guilt and shame and sorrow and anguish and anger, all of which I am still dealing with more than four years after being discharged from the hospital.

Months later, I invite Clare to be my date at a gala benefit for the Preeclampsia Foundation. She immediately begins saving up her "giving money," that portion of her weekly allowance that's designated for helping others, whether a nonprofit organization or the man with severe burns who regularly panhandles on Pearl Street. Who receives Clare's contribution is always her decision to make.

We fly to Minneapolis, and Clare walks into the banquet hall dressed in a black velvet dress with a puffy white tulle skirt, one hand in mine and the other clutching four one-dollar bills. A quick glance around the room tells me she's the only child in attendance, but I'm not concerned. She's earned her place at this event every bit as much as any of the older attendees. After signing in, I scout the room for Eleni, whom I'd met a month ago during one of my blood donation talks in her home state of California. I find her, we hug, and I introduce her to Clare, who proudly hands Eleni her four dollars of giving money as a donation to the foundation.

Eleni introduces us to the hosts of the banquet, Jaime and Joe, both in their late twenties, perhaps early thirties. I've already read about their ordeal, how a year earlier their daughter, Grace, was born prematurely due to preeclampsia, weighing less than two pounds. At five days old, Grace went into cardiac arrest, and Joe watched as a doctor used his thumb to perform chest compressions during CPR. Grace went into cardiac arrest four more times before passing away several days later. In the following months, Jaime's grief morphed into a profound desire to do something, to prevent other couples from having to go through a similar experience. She launched Saving Grace: A Night of Hope, not knowing that it would become the annual gala benefit for the Preeclampsia Foundation, not knowing how many people it would connect, encourage, and inspire—not the least among them me.

Clare and I walk among the tables of silent auction items, bidding on things that I know she's interested in only because she's caught up in the excitement of being at a big fancy party. When the dinner chimes ring, we snake our way through the banquet hall to find our assigned table. The man and woman seated next to us are from rural Iowa and maybe ten years older than me. Quiet and distanced from the festivities, John and Brenda seem a bit out of place among the energetic thirty-something friends of Jaime and Joe who dominate the gathering. Making small talk, I ask about their connection to this cause and then listen, dumbfounded, as John tells me the story of their twenty-five-year-old daughter, Shelly, who developed preeclampsia ten months earlier. The details of her story—the sudden onset of the disease, the liver failure, the bleeding—are eerily similar to mine, but with one key difference. A week after the premature delivery of her baby, Shelly died. In gaining their first grandchild, John and Brenda lost their first child. Like Jaime and Joe, Shelly's parents decided they would do what they could to prevent others from going through a similar experience. They came to the event to present the foundation with a check for $1,200, proceeds from a walkathon they'd recently hosted in honor of Shelly.

As I look about the room, listen to several couples share their stories at the podium, and take in the startling statistics about preeclampsia, I realize I no longer feel alone or peculiar or at fault for having had such a dramatic case of the disease. I sense the affinity I share with this room full of strangers, many of us bound by a common affliction, many of us trying to do what we can to prevent others from joining our sisterhood.

When the event ends, Clare and I return to our hotel room with a bellman in tow, pushing a luggage cart piled high with *Cat in the Hat* dolls, the Batman gift set, a bin of art supplies, and an enormous Lego set that the event emcee mentioned during her remarks, stating, "I had my eye on those Legos, but some kid boxed me out during the final thirty seconds of bidding." On our way to the airport the next morning, I ask the taxi driver to stop downtown at a seafood supplier so I can pick up the case of fresh Alaskan king crab legs I won during the live auction. One week later, and sick of crabmeat, I begin making plans for next year's Saving Grace. Despite having never planned a formal event other than my junior prom, I agreed to chair the 2006 gala benefit in San Francisco.

I have no idea how to go about securing major sponsors, contracting with a hotel, or getting people to attend, but everything changes the day my dentist prescribes Valium. I'm scheduled to have the mercury removed from my teeth, and he knows I'm extremely nervous about the procedure. Making me promise not to drive, he tells me to take one pill the night before and another the morning of my appointment.

After taking the first Valium of my life, I crawl into Clare's upper bunk bed for one of our weekly mommy-daughter sleepovers. Clare falls asleep almost immediately, but not me. Feeling warm and woozy, I use the glow of the night-light to take in the years of memories stored in my daughter's bedroom. I still love the purple walls and purple carpeting I added when we first moved in, when Clare was too young to tell me that her first favorite color would be Buzz Lightyear green, not lavender, violet, plum, or any other shade of purple. Hanging from the ceiling on fishing line are the yellow, green, and purple felt stars I took hours to pick out at the baby store in San Francisco when I was pregnant. Mixed among them are the half-dozen ceramic fairies Jeff's parents gave Clare during the themed party we threw for her in Michigan, the party in which we all dressed in brightly colored tights, nylon wings, and outfits that reflected the type of fairies we were: the Dog Fairy, the Fire Fairy, the Fairy Godmother. The origami crane mobiles that Clare's preschool teacher made for her fourth and fifth birthdays dangle from opposite sides of the room, illuminated by dozens of small plastic glow-in-the-dark adhesive stars. Several poster-size photo collages made by my mother-in-law hang on one of the bedroom walls and depict every phase of my daughter's life, from my pregnancy to her current age: pictures of Clare picking apples, doing yoga, dyeing Easter eggs. On another wall is a framed eight-by-ten photo of Jeff and me, the one we snapped holding the camera at arm's length right after I stepped off the plane from Paris, the last photo taken before I was pregnant hours later. Purple celestial curtains made by her "Aunt" Jane adorn the windows facing the foothills. And a bookcase in the corner holds favorite books, like those by Lemony Snicket, the Gaspard and Lisa series, and *My Monster Mama Loves Me So*, as well as her snow globe collection and several framed photos of Spike, who passed away four months earlier.

Lying in the bunk bed, I savor the mementos of my daughter's life, symbols that might easily have never existed had fate and fortune and medical expertise not conspired to save her life. I am both profoundly grateful that Clare and I survived and profoundly saddened by all the stories of death due to preeclampsia that I've recently encountered. My grief and gratitude ignite a desire in me to host the most inspired Saving Grace event possible, an homage to those who've lost their lives and a promise of hope for future generations of mothers.

And then it hits me: *Weldon.* Of course! Weldon!

I climb down the bunk-bed ladder and pad downstairs to my home office, unaware that my feelings of inspiration and goodwill are likely prompted by the Valium I took an hour ago. I sit at my computer and tap out an e-mail message with the subject header *Please Say Yes!* In the body of the e-mail I say that I've committed to chairing a gala benefit for the Preeclampsia Foundation and that *the only thing I want for Christmas this year is for you to agree to be my co-chair.* I click "Send," and off goes the first e-mail I've ever sent to the chairman of the board of Johnson & Johnson, a man whose responsibilities include overseeing more than 220 companies worldwide. Pleased with my brainstorm, I turn out the lights in my office and climb back in bed with Clare, giving not one thought to my impending dental work or the audacity of going right to the top of the Johnson & Johnson chain of command.

The following morning, I awaken and lie in bed trying to decipher foggy thoughts I'm having, something about Bill Weldon and Saving Grace and e-mail. *Was that a dream?* I slip out of bed, careful not to wake Clare, and make my way to the computer. Nope, not a dream. *Oh well.* Either he'll have a sense of humor about my e-mail or not. Any negative consequence to my drug-induced request will be nothing compared to getting a transjugular liver biopsy. I pop another Valium and go to the dentist's office.

That afternoon, I receive an e-mail from a woman named Linda Gallo. *Mr. Weldon is currently traveling out of the country,* it reads. *I'll see that he receives your request concerning the gala benefit.* What Linda doesn't mention in her reply is that pre-eclampsia nearly killed her best friend several decades earlier. Two days later, she writes to say that her boss would be "delighted" to co-chair the event with me. I know this means that I'll still be managing all the logistics, but Johnson & Johnson will write a sizable check to the cause, and the fact that Bill Weldon is involved will bring additional sponsors and guaranteed attendance.

Eleven months later, at the Mark Hopkins Hotel on top of Nob Hill in San Francisco, Clare attends her second Saving Grace benefit. Jeff emcees, looking smart in his new black suit. I share my story, looking slimmer—fourteen pounds lost to the stress of the planning—in my new cocktail dress. And Clare, who requested a part in the show as soon as she learned that both Jeff and I would be on stage, stands before four hundred adults and sings the simple nondenominational blessing that she and her fellow first-graders sing everyday at snack time.

Bill Weldon, fresh off a flight from Japan, makes good on his promise to cohost the event. Mayor Gavin Newsom stops by, one of several appearances he's scheduled to make tonight. Eleni shares an update on the foundation, and founder Anne Garrett helps recognize some of the leaders in preeclampsia research. Jazz violinist Regina Carter, an old friend of Jeff's who weeks earlier was awarded a MacArthur Foundation "genius grant," came from New York to provide the music for a slideshow of preeclampsia stories that are both heartbreaking and hopeful. Regina plays "Amazing Grace," the same song she played for me in the ICU six years earlier when she was in town for a concert and stopped by the hospital at Jeff's request. Just as important to me as the luminaries on the stage are some of the many friends, new and old, who make up the audience. Jaime and Joe have come from Minnesota with their recently adopted baby, Brian. My former neighbor Katherine sponsored two tables and has brought her extended family with her. George, the kidney doctor who copresented with me at the TED-MED conference two years ago, is here, as is Kelly, a heart-transplant patient and world-renowned mountain climber, whose story I share regularly during my blood donation talks. Three tables are filled with nurses, several of whom cared for me while I was sick, all of whom used my hotel suite as a dressing room prior to the event. Dusa is here, and she gives me another healing crystal. One of my blood donors, Adam, brought his framed Certificate of Thanks from Clare with him, proudly showing it to me as we hug and have our photo taken together. Mike, the president of the blood center two hours away, gives me a beautifully packaged pie, a humorous reminder of the time I emceed his employee appreciation event and decided to go off script and smash a pie in his face. Also in the bakery box is a donation for $1,000, which brings tears to my eyes for not the first time tonight.

By the time the banquet ends, I am thoroughly spent. The effects of consuming only five bites of a quesadilla and three Cokes all day, combined with my anxiety of wanting to pull off a successful event, have taken their toll. Back in our hotel room, I leave my stockings and pricey dress in a heap on the floor and curl up on the couch wearing a hotel bathrobe. With a double order of room service lasagna on my lap and a glass of chardonnay in my hand, I laugh and talk with old friends, all crammed into our suite for the private after-party. At two in the morning, the last guest departs, and Jeff and I join Clare in bed, where she's been asleep for hours. The next morning, my lead volunteer, Jess Swann, calls with the final tallies for the night. Saving Grace raised more than $265,000, and the team of two dozen volunteers, mostly former work colleagues and friends, has pulled off the largest fundraiser in the foundation's history. One of those volunteers is Lisa Bloch, who in one month will become pregnant with her first child.

Seven weeks before her due date, Lisa calls my cell phone. After the success of the Patient-Donor Reunion, she had asked me to emcee a similar event a year later for Meghan, a college student who needed 987 pints of blood, so I assume Lisa's calling about another speaking opportunity.

"Lisa Bloch!" I say. "What's up, girl?"

"You are really *not* going to believe this," she says, sounding slightly woozy.

"Try me."

"You know how I'm always saying that you're my role model and I want to be like you when I grow up?"

"Um, no, but go ahead."

"Well, I think I should be more careful about what I wish for. I have preeclampsia."

"No!"

"Yes. And I'm actually at the hospital now, the same one that treated you. I got diagnosed about an hour ago and they're wheeling me up to Labor & Delivery now."

"You have got to be kidding!"

"I wish I was."

"Who's treating you?"

"Dr. Main. He's supposed to be one of the best."

"Well, he was called in on my case, so I'd have to agree."

"Same high-risk OB? I really need to slow down on emulating you."

"No, what you really need to do is pick a new role model."

Weeks later, back at home with her new baby girl, Lisa shares with me the details that led to Zoe's premature C-section birth. She tells me how she went to the emergency room with severe upper abdominal pain—a classic sign of preeclampsia; she was misdiagnosed with a pulled muscle and sent home with Percocet. When Lisa had blinding headaches two days later, she was misdiagnosed a second time and told to take an extra Percocet for her "migraines." Again, another symptom of preeclampsia was overlooked. When Lisa began seeing stars—a third symptom of preeclampsia—she thought back on all the talks of mine she'd attended, all the times she'd heard me rattle off the signs and symptoms of preeclampsia, and the information she'd learned while volunteering for the Saving Grace event. Returning to the hospital, she shared her symptoms with one of the antepartum nurses, who immediately phoned Dr. Main. Later, after baby Zoe's five-weeks-premature delivery, Lisa was told that had she not come in, she would've likely gone into kidney failure and her baby would've probably died in utero.

Ever since connecting with the Preeclampsia Foundation, I found myself repeating their mantra during my talks: *Know the symptoms. Trust yourself.* After a while, it sounded almost clichéd to me. Until Lisa. She knew the symptoms and, ultimately, allowed her instinct to override the misdiagnoses. One woman, one baby saved by the creation of a patient-advocacy organization, a sisterhood of those wanting to prevent others from experiencing the losses they have.

One woman.

One baby.

40

"AN ELECTRIC GUITAR!" Clare squeals, her six-year-old astonishment infectious, her belief in Santa rock solid. She rushes across the living room in her rumpled pajamas and giant dog slippers, and drops to her knees in front of the black-and-white child-size Fender leaning against the amplifier. "Santa brought me an electric guitar!" Jeff and I exchange glances that say *Yep, we did good.*

Since attending her first Saving Grace gala benefit, when she spotted the electric guitar signed by Paul McCartney and was disappointed that I refused to bid on it during the live auction, Clare has expressed an interest in getting her own, at times to the point of badgering. She added acoustic guitar to her weekly piano lessons but was never fully satisfied with the gentle nature of its sound. When she sat down last night to write up her wish list for Santa, I already knew what would be on it: Silly String, a disco ball, anything Hannah Montana, and an electric guitar. Jeff and I had already decided that this would be the year we'd let a mythical fat man in a fuzzy red jumpsuit take credit for delivering her long-cherished desire in the quiet of the night.

The innocence of Clare's belief in all things magical—Santa, the Easter Bunny, the Tooth Fairy—remains strong. Many of her classmates at the small contemplative-education school that she attends are singletons, so the chances of older siblings spoiling the fun are minimal. As far as I'm concerned, there's plenty of time to learn more about life's hardships and unfairness. For now I want to fuel the wonder in Clare's life.

"That Santa," I say. "He sure is a great guy."

"Sure is," Jeff adds, rubbing his freshly shaven scalp.

"Does it still feel weird?" I ask him. I've noticed the frequency with which he runs his hand over the top of his head since asking me to shave it recently with the same shears that removed the remnants of my own hair six years earlier. It's as if he's been experiencing "phantom hair," like an amputee who has the sensation of the missing limb still being present.

"Actually, it feels good. But it's not exactly the best hairdo for winter in Boulder."

"Perfect for Sudan, though."

"Dad, when do you have to leave?" Clare asks, disengaging from her new guitar.

"We've got a few more hours," Jeff says. "No rush."

He takes Clare's guitar in hand and breaks into a goofy imitation of Jimi Hendrix, clearly moving the focus away from his imminent departure. Then, setting the guitar aside, he says, "Hey, let's look in our stockings!"

Clare rifles through an array of candies and stickers and action figures from her purple Christmas stocking, using her free arm to shoo our two poodle puppies away as they clamber over one another in hopes of snatching a treat. Gigham and Duke joined our family last February, and while certainly no replacement for my beloved Spike, their exuberance has soothed the sting of her death a year and a half ago. When Clare reaches the three cans of Silly String stuffed into the bottom of her stocking, her excitement is almost on a par with discovering the electric guitar.

Jeff and I move to the kitchen, where he brews a pot of coffee and I prepare bagels and lox. Mom and John arrive from their home two minutes away, and we all gather in the living room to watch Clare as she eagerly tears Sponge Bob holiday wrapping paper off puzzles, a Magic 8 Ball, origami paper, and an assortment of what we call "stupid humor" movies. We push through the festivities with a slight undertone of urgency, knowing that there are still several tasks we need to complete before I take Jeff to the airport this afternoon, yet trying hard not to dampen the fun for Clare.

"So do you feel ready for the trip?" John asks Jeff.

"Ready as I'll ever be," Jeff says. "Things really came together these last couple weeks."

He and John walk over to the dining room, where most of Jeff's gear is packed in duffle bags and backpacks, and he points out his various supplies: camera equipment for photography and videography; an enormous canvas bag of first-aid and medical supplies purchased in bulk from Costco—a last-minute inspiration of mine; and gifts for the villagers: candies, marbles, and English dictionaries for the children, scarves for the women, dominos and cribbage for the men. One backpack holds all of the clothing, netting, vitamins and medications, energy bars, and toiletries that Jeff will need for the entire four-week trip.

Sending my husband off to war-torn areas of a developing country in sub-Saharan Africa to drill water wells was never an intention of mine, nor something Jeff had ever imagined himself doing. We both grew up in small middle-class towns in which matters of global poverty were something talked about only in public service announcements on television. Though I've been a supporter of Save the Children since I was a college student, even that felt safe and distant, the hardships of the people assisted by my monthly donation brought to life only through the occasional newsletter. But five years ago, when Jeff and I met the Lost Boys shortly after they resettled in Denver, our eyes and hearts were opened to the greater suffering of the world in a very direct way. The kindness of strangers—blood donors in particular—had helped us through our toughest challenge in life, so it felt only natural to offer that same kindness to these Sudanese strangers who were still going through theirs.

Over time, Jeff's and my relationship with the Lost Boys shifted from that of parents to that of friends, the focus of our interactions from job applications and cooking lessons to college graduations and citizenship ceremonies. Clare delighted in introducing the Lost Boys as "my Sudanese brothers," or dyeing Easter eggs for them, or hanging out in their apartment while Jeff fixed the latest technical problem with the second-hand computers we had given them. Since the beginning, many of them consistently expressed their desire to return to their homeland when there was peace and to help rebuild. We promised to help them do just that—*when there was peace* being the imperative condition.

That day came sooner than expected when, in January 2005, a peace treaty was signed between the Sudanese government and the SPLA—the Sudanese People's Liberation Army, which had been gaining strength over the years as it rose up against the decades-long campaign of government-sanctioned attacks in the south. The time had come to make good on our promise, even though our level of debt had increased considerably with Jeff's return to school full time.

Once more, we put pen to paper and wrote an appeal for help from our friends. Working with Panther, one of our original "sons," we teamed up with a local nonprofit, Project Education Sudan, which was founded by another Lost Boy and a Denver couple. Their goal is to build schools, so we committed to drilling one water well at each school location. Another Boulder resident who'd been deeply involved with the Lost Boys is an electrician, and he and his Sudanese "son," Lual, committed to bringing solar-powered electricity to the villages. Still another offered to underwrite a commercial grain grinder, which would allow girls to attend school instead of spending the day grinding the family's grain by hand. A true grassroots effort was under way and, soon enough, an expedition team consisting of six Americans and six Lost Boys was formed.

In March of that year, deep into my national speaking tour for blood donation, I emceed a five-hour employee appreciation event for the nonprofit blood center in Sacramento. At the end of the celebration, the CEO, Mike Fuller, called me back to the stage to thank me. I accepted the plaque he handed to me and presumed we were finished. But then Mike began telling the audience about the Lost Boys and Jeff's and my letter campaign to raise money for water wells in the remote areas of southern Sudan. He pulled an envelope from his suit jacket and presented me with a check for $8,000, compliments of the employees of BloodSource.

I stared, dumbfounded, at the audience of roughly 500 people, and for the first time in my five-year speaking tour, I simply could not find words. Afterward I walked back to my hotel, cell phone to my ear, and told Jeff what had happened, now unable to stop the words from coming. Neither of us could believe that a California-based blood center would extend its lifesaving efforts to include providing clean water for remote villages halfway around the world. On the other hand, ever since my illness we'd been recognizing more and more examples of synchronicity in our lives, and we'd come to trust that the unlikeliest of connections could often develop into the most profound ones.

"Clare! Time to go!" I yell to my daughter, who is upstairs in her bedroom jamming on her electric guitar and singing into a microphone. *This is a song I wrote myself!* I hear her wail over the jarring sounds of the guitar. *And I didn't get any help!* Pause. *This is a song I wrote myself!* Pause. *And it's all about me!* She's been singing these same lyrics over and over for the past hour, no doubt enjoying her inaugural performance as a singer-songwriter in front of the full-length mirror. At one point, I was laughing so hard I called my sister Karen in Pennsylvania and held the phone out toward the ruckus so she too could enjoy Clare's new rocker persona.

Jeff and I load the car with his luggage and drive Clare to her friend Poet's house to play, thereby diffusing the intensity of a drawn-out airport farewell. Arriving at Denver International, we meet up with five other Americans, all dressed in lightweight outdoor adventure gear, and Panther, dressed as if he's headed to a nightclub. Despite the crippling heat and humidity they're bound to encounter once on the ground in Africa, this is Panther's homecoming, and his wardrobe choice says he's determined to look his best. I tease him about making the rest of the team look like slobs and he laughs easily at the humor. It's hard to believe that just five Christmases ago, he sat in our living room with seven other Sudanese, all awkwardly pulling new underpants and toiletries from their stockings and looking mildly embarrassed by the personal nature of the gifts.

The other five Lost Boys going on this "reunification" trip have already left on earlier flights, so the entire team will meet up in Nairobi before boarding another plane to Lokichoggio, Kenya, about thirty miles from the border of Sudan. There they'll board the smaller plane they've chartered to take them into the remote backcountry, where they'll touch down on a landing strip that was recently created by villagers beating the ground with sticks for this very flight.

For two hours, we repack duffle bags and equipment cases on the airport floor near the check-in counter, redistributing the weight of the tools and building supplies to meet airline regulations. Then I hug Jeff hard, holding onto him with the full knowledge that we're about to have our longest separation since I backpacked through Europe right before getting pregnant, before we faced the most pronounced turning point in our lives. This feels like another of those turning points, as if we're about to enter another new arena in this adventure called life: that of the global community.

Over the following weeks, I keep my cell phone close at hand,
uncertain as to when the next call will come in from Jeff on the
satellite phone we rented for the trip. The communications are
brief and filled with the crackling of static, and I'm never sure
how long we'll have before the line is inevitably dropped. During Jeff's first call from within the borders of Sudan, I'm strolling the aisles of Target with Clare and realize I don't have any
paper in my purse. She and I run through the store to the office
supplies section where I grab a notebook and begin furiously
taking notes as Jeff conveys the latest news, which I'll then type
up and forward to the forty or so people on the e-mail list:
other spouses and friends and Lost Boys, all as eager to hear
the latest reports as I am now. He tells me how hundreds of
villagers turned out to greet them when their chartered plane
landed in the bush, how amazing it is to be living in thatched
huts among the people, all of whom have been generous beyond
their means—the cooking of a coveted family cow to celebrate
their arrival, or the gift of one warm bottle of beer for Jeff each
night as the meal is prepared.

He tells me of the dire lack of medical care in these remote
villages and how a Christian missionary from Omaha, Ne-
braska, has been managing the local first-aid needs for several
months with no training other than what she'd learned watching medical dramas on TV back home. In speaking with her, he
learned that she'd recently run out of all medical supplies and
when the villagers, some of whom had walked for days to get
help, asked her what they would do now, she'd told them not
to worry, that God would provide. And then, as if in a burst of
cosmic irony, my atheist husband showed up days later, a huge
duffle bag of medical supplies in hand. I laugh out loud at that
one, and Jeff tells me that even he and his new friend from
Omaha saw the humor in the situation.

On another call, Jeff tells me how he and David, the electrician, found bats clinging to the low-hung roof of their hut

each night and how they tried shooing them out with sticks but it didn't work. Finally, one of the elders walked into their hut and loudly clapped his hands, which sent the bats fleeing. On another night, he says, he had relaxed enough to exchange his army-surplus combat boots for flip-flops while sitting in the dark by the fire, only to have that be the night he came face-to-toe with a scorpion when he went to the bathroom hut to relieve himself. He laughs as he recounts how his body was instantly flooded with adrenaline, and though scared out of his wits, he instinctively stomped the scorpion to mush while barking *Die, motherfucker, die!* over and over again.

Through these calls I learn about the progress of the water wells as Jeff and Panther work with the drilling team from Uganda, which includes several Sudanese men, among them Panther's uncle. He tells me of the unexpected frustrations they've encountered and overcome: the hours of debate among village elders regarding specifically where within the community each well would be located, or the difficulty of drilling the full 200-foot depth required for a sustainable water supply, or the need for a stick fence to be erected around each well so the roaming cattle won't damage it. He also tells me how the local children gathered at the site of the first well-drilling and sat patiently for hours with worn and dirty plastic containers, waiting for water to appear. When the drilling rig finally hit the aquifer and fresh uncontaminated water shot out of the ground, the jubilance and dancing and splashing of all those children now crammed around the borehole was almost too much for Jeff to take. This is the first fresh water in the area, and thousands of locals will no longer have to walk half a day for stagnant river water, or a full day or more for fresh water from the only other pump within miles. Sitting in my home office halfway around the world, I replay the scene over and over in my mind as tears slide down my cheeks.

Days later, the group has moved on to another location, where Panther at last got to reunite with his mother after nineteen years, many of which he spent not knowing if she had even survived the war. Jeff tells me how they drove deep into the bush, following the cryptic directions they'd been given. When their Jeep finally came to a halt, word of their arrival spread quickly throughout the network of huts, and soon one of Panther's aunties was running hysterically across the brush toward him. Shortly after she smothered him in hugs, his mother arrived, so tiny and frail that Panther had to bend down to embrace her. Jeff tells me that Panther was clearly as shaken as his mother, and that the two of them had to step back, even turn away momentarily, as if in disbelief or shock over the long-awaited reunion. I sense that Jeff is shaken too, the thought of being separated from your own child for so long an inconceivable notion to him. He tells me how they later sat in a hut together and Jeff presented gifts to Panther's family members, and in exchange, Panther interpreted as his mother offered blessings and gratitude to Jeff for being both a friend and a father to her child, for bringing him back home to her. As I hear the details of this story in particular—a mother and child reunited—the lump in my throat grows. I realize that despite the vast differences in who we are and how we live, Panther's mother and I share a unifying theme. Two women, separated from their children. Two women, reconnected with their children. And intricately involved in both scenarios is Jeff. Steadfast, loyal Jeff.

During Jeff's last week in Sudan, I take Clare with me to several speaking engagements in Florida, and when my work is finished, we stay a few days more at a hotel on the beach, my thinly veiled effort at preempting any sadness she might otherwise feel over her dad being away. Clare and I share a mutual love of all beaches, all waves, all sand, and my plan is clearly working. She remains upbeat even though this is the longest she's been away from Jeff since she was a newborn and living with my brother's family. One morning as we begin our daily stroll along the shoreline, Clare tells me she really, really wants to find a sand dollar today.

"Set an intention," I say. "Just put your wish out there to the ocean and the sky and whatever else might be listening that you'd sure like to have a sand dollar."

She closes her eyes and concentrates, her little feet sinking deeper into the soft wet sand at the water's edge. When she opens her eyes again, we walk hand in hand, me gazing at the distant shoreline, enjoying the sun on my face, her intently looking at the ground before her, searching for that sand dollar. We make it to our usual halfway point and begin walking back in the direction of the hotel, Clare still searching, seeking, showing signs of frustration, then resignation. We're almost to the wooden walkway that leads to our hotel when a woman in her retirement years stops Clare and asks, "Would you like to have this?" She stretches her arm toward Clare and unclenches her hand to reveal a perfect sand dollar in her palm.

"Wow!" Clare says. "Thank you!" Beaming, she gently takes the sand dollar and continues staring at it even as we say our goodbyes to the older woman. When we're out of earshot, I lean toward Clare.

"Well, what do you know?" I say. "Looks like you made your wish come true!"

"But I didn't find it," she says. "It was given to me."

"Sometimes, Clare, the things we want most come to us in the unlikeliest of ways."

Returning to Boulder the following day, Clare and I prepare for Jeff's homecoming. She makes a giant poster board sign to hold up in the international waiting area at the airport, and she digs through our party supply box to find Hawaiian leis, noisemakers, and party horns—necessary accoutrements for any occasion, according to my daughter. We order helium balloons and pick them up on our way to the airport, bringing enough to share with the other spouses and friends who've come to await the team's return. Clare distributes the supplies, and as I watch her I'm impressed with how calm she is, that she's made it the full length of Jeff's trip without any emotional meltdowns.

We hover near the sliding doors that separate the customs area from the waiting area, and Clare strains to find Jeff among the throngs going through customs each time the sliding doors open. She's already told me she's going to give him the biggest hug he's ever had in his life, but when the doors part once more and it's Jeff who steps through them, my daughter crumples to the floor in a flood of tears. With her head in her hands, she cries so hard she can't even make eye contact with the father she's missed so deeply she had to hide those feelings from even herself. Jeff leans across the bar that keeps loved ones from crowding the exit, gives me a kiss, then reaches down and scoops up Clare in his arms, and we three cling to one another in a private group hug.

Within our little family we have each gone away for an extended period: Clare to live with Tim and Dede, me to illness and loss of consciousness, and Jeff to Sudan. And perhaps it is these fantastical journeys that strengthen our sense of unity. We each went away. But we each came back. Whether separated through war or illness or adventure, in families there is always the hope of reunion, the joy of reconnecting. Like the Lost Boys to surviving family members they'd not seen in almost two decades. Like Clare's return to San Francisco after my release from the hospital. Like Jeff's homecoming now.

41

IT IS SEVEN YEARS since my illness, and I'm now on my fifth primary-care physician in hopes of finding one who might shed light on why I'm still having residual health issues and, more importantly, what I might do to advance my recovery. After my initial intake visit last week, I return for a blood sample, the simple extraction of two small vials of blood from my body. Arriving at the doctor's office, I explain to the receptionist that because of my bleeding history, I'll need the most experienced phlebotomist on staff to do my blood draw, as my veins are no longer cooperative. I'll also require the use of a "butterfly" needle, the smallest size available, typically reserved for pediatric use. I'm friendly but firm in my request, and soon I'm led into the back room, where two nurses greet me.

"This is Tiffany," the older woman says. "She's new to our office and she'll be drawing your blood today."

"You're *new?*" I ask.

"My second day," she says, her voice bubbly in a way that does nothing to inspire confidence. I look more closely at Tiffany and estimate her age to be twenty-four at most.

"She's got lots of experience, don't you worry," the other nurse says.

I'm unconvinced, and I know my trepidation is showing. I've been through several unsuccessful blood draws since the illness and have learned that DIC, the bleeding disorder triggered by my preeclampsia, often weakens the vascular system irreversibly.

"That is not a butterfly needle," I say, noticing the tray of sterile supplies.

"This one should be just fine," the older nurse says. "Besides, those butterfly needles take so long. We'll have you out of here in no time."

My breath catches in my throat and I can feel my neck constrict into my shoulders. *Don't be a wimp,* I silently chide myself. Turning my head away, I close my eyes and will myself to be brave. Tiffany jabs my arm and the pain is immediate.

"Oops, didn't quite get it," she says. She jabs a second time, again missing her mark. Switching arms, she tries again, all the while chirping on about this and that. I refuse to engage in conversation, no longer concerned with being congenial. All my energy is focused on holding back tears that I sense are connected to so much more than a few painful thrusts of a needle. After Tiffany's fifth failed attempt at drawing my blood, I reach my breaking point and begin sobbing uncontrollably.

"I told the receptionist I needed the most experienced phlebotomist on staff!" I say through tears and snot, my voice choking every few words. "I told her I had vascular issues! I told her I needed a butterfly needle! Didn't she tell you? Why doesn't anyone *listen?*"

Tiffany doesn't say a word, but simply steps away, shell-shocked, as the older nurse moves in to take over, handing me a box of tissues.

"Let's get you that butterfly needle," she says, rubbing my back. I continue crying as the senior nurse inserts a smaller needle, easily, into a vein on the top of my right hand and within minutes has drawn the necessary blood. As soon as the cotton ball is taped over the small puncture wound, I walk out without so much as goodbye.

In the waiting area, several patients look up from their magazines to see the woman who caused the disturbance. I hasten past, slowing only to glare at the receptionist, hoping my tearstained face and blank expression convey my disdain for her. Pushing open the heavy lobby doors, I know I'll never return to this office again.

Once inside my car, I sit in the parking lot, the car idling, for over half an hour, as I grab tissue after tissue from a full box, crying, blowing my nose, pounding the steering wheel, and talking to myself. *Listen, damn it! Why is it so hard to just listen?* Memories of the ICU choke me—of needles and arm restraints; of people telling me that something won't hurt, just a small pinch, that's all, that the pain I feel isn't actually pain. They said these things over and over again, paying no attention to my objections, my sobbing. And now, all these years later, they're *still* not listening!

Studies posted on the Preeclampsia Foundation Web site describe the discovery of Post-Traumatic Stress Disorder in survivors of severe preeclampsia. While recently reading about that research, it never occurred to me that *I* might be one of those women whose emotional wounds run deeper than her physical ones. Clearly, Tiffany pierced a layer of dormant trauma, and I'm beginning to understand why some of my emotional reactions seem disproportionate or inappropriate to the situation. Why, for instance, all television dramas involving the loss of a baby or child, regardless of how amateurish the production is, tap a wellspring of tears from deep within me. Or why, to the contrary, when several doctors familiar with my medical history say things like "You should be dead" as a way to underscore the severity of my case, I wave them off with a humorous quip.

I now understand that it had been too soon to explore any scars other than those visible to the eye: ten on my abdomen, seven around my neck. Slowly, tentatively, I begin healing not just the physical ailments, but the emotional ones as well. And in so doing, I allow myself to shed the tears of grief I felt but could not express all those years ago, while conscious and angry and wracked with guilt in the hospital.

In the spring of 2000, one day before Jeff showed up with a bouquet of roses for his pregnant wife, my mother-in-law mailed me a book. This in itself wasn't unusual. Bev knows I love books, and she and my father-in-law often send them as birthday and anniversary gifts. What *was* unusual was that there was no special occasion for this gift. She just felt like it, she'd tell me later. And even more unusual was her choice of books: *For Whom the Bell Tolls.*

Once Bev heard the news of my rapid decline following Clare's birth, she panicked about the book's imminent arrival and phoned to have someone intercept the package. Months later, we would laugh about the irony of sending a book whose primary theme is *death* to a woman who—unbeknownst to all of us—was about to face her own. "What an odd coincidence," Jeff said to me on more than one occasion.

But was it?

Clearly, my mother-in-law didn't have conscious knowledge about the medical catastrophe I was about to face, but could her act of sending that particular book on that particular day have been some sort of accidental premonition? And what of the other strange things that, in hindsight, seemed to hold greater significance than I granted them as they occurred?

What of Spike's behavior on the day of Clare's birth, her refusal to leave my side even for her usual morning walk with Jeff? I've heard stories of dogs that can detect cancer in a body and dogs that know when seizures are about to overtake their human guardians. Why not a dog that can sense the onset of severe preeclampsia? Is it really too much of a stretch to think that Spike was trying to warn me, protect me? Am I to brush off her unusual behavior as coincidence?

What of the psychic friend of my mother's who, early in my pregnancy, told Mom she "saw" an allergic reaction happening at Clare's birth? Seven months later, I'd hear my obstetrician describe preeclampsia as an "allergic reaction" between mother and baby as she signed the orders for my emergency C-section. Is it possible that a disease that's often undetected or misdiagnosed by trained medical professionals could be foreseen by someone I'd never met?

And what am I to think of Monica? Should I simply ignore what she said to me five months before I became pregnant? In February 1999, I was in New York on business and decided to get together with an astrologer friend who lived in the city. "You thinking of getting pregnant?" Monica asked me. I told her no, giving her the same explanation I would give Mia during our Barcelona picnic four months later: Jeff's ambivalent and I'm not ready. "Well, your chart shows a baby coming into your life in May of 2000," she said. "If it's not yours, perhaps it'll be a new niece or nephew." *Doubtful*, I thought. All my siblings, in-laws included, were finished having children.

Six months later, when my obstetrician calculated my due date, I remembered that Monica had said something about a baby, so I dug through my files until I found the notes from our meeting. *Aha!* my inner skeptic thought, triumphant. She may have gotten the baby part right, but she was off by two months. Clare was due to arrive in late March, not May. And yet when Dede brought Clare home to live with Jeff and me, when we were finally reunited as a family and my sister-in-law left for the airport, her duties as interim mother fulfilled, the date was the first of May.

Even recently, I heard from Peter, who left ICU work shortly after helping save my life to become a primary-care nurse practitioner. He e-mailed me from Moscow, where he works for the American embassy, to tell me of a dream he'd had while I was unconscious and not expected to live. *Dearest*, he wrote, *I*

must tell you that I had a very strong dream about you during
hospitalization. I was somewhere doing something with someone—
another typical dream—when suddenly I saw you seated at a table
with Jeff, laughing. "Lauren! How could this be?" I asked. "I mean,
you died!" You looked at me, smiling, and said, "Oh Peter, that was
such a long time ago!" I awoke and it was so reassuring. I really
wanted you to live. And you did!"

Wishful thinking? Or had Peter tapped into some well of
consciousness that allowed him to glimpse the future, encouraging him to go back into the ICU and give me his best for
another sixteen-hour shift, to take comfort in knowing that it
was still possible to create a positive outcome in an otherwise
hopeless situation?

Years before I went through this inconceivable adventure, I
struggled with the concept of fate versus free will, often wondering *Which is it?* Are we puppets in a play whose ending has
already been written? Or are we the authors of our own stories,
with nothing predestined? My friend Andrew once told me he
believed that life included *both* destiny and free will. "Fate is
that you must climb that mountain," he said. "Free will is how
you choose to do it." This theory resonated with me, that two
opposing concepts could peacefully coexist. But theory and application are two different things, and theory, I've learned, can
evaporate in an instant when its application involves excruciating physical and emotional pain.

The desire to dissect my illness, to pull apart every aspect of
this remarkable and hellish turning point in my life, grew as my
physical recovery progressed. Could I have prevented this? Or
was it an unavoidable calamity? What if I'd eaten less Taco Bell
during my pregnancy? What if I'd paid closer attention to my
symptoms? What if I'd picked a different OB? What if I'd been
more attentive in the all-day birthing class? *What if Jeff hadn't*
brought me those roses?

Ultimately, I settled on this interpretation: The experience of nearly dying is one of the mountains that make up my fate in life. The decisions and changes I've made since leaving the hospital are how I've chosen to climb that mountain.

While I struggled to make sense of what had happened to me, others seemed to have their own interpretations of my experience. When I was lying unconscious in the ICU, one friend wrote that she was certain this was a sign that I should accept Jesus into my life and become a Christian. But how could she be so certain that facing my death was a sign that Jesus—or *any* prophet, god, or spiritual entity for that matter—had launched a personal recruitment campaign for my soul? Ironically, my new-found relationship with mortality has made me even more comfortable with my own *lack* of certainty in matters of the spirit.

Another well-intentioned friend suggested that I had a karmic debt to repay, as if all those blood transfusions that saved my life were hanging over my head as a big reminder that payment was now due on some cosmic invoice with my name written across the top. I rejected her perspective as well. The gift of all those blood donors who decided, for whatever reason, to give an hour of their time to save the life of a woman they'd never met, was just that—a gift. And true gifts incur no debt.

Then there was the outlook of my buddy Kev, a former publishing colleague turned shamanic healer, who—shortly after I'd moved to Boulder—asked me, "Why do you suppose you chose to create your illness? What was its purpose in your life?" At the time I was as bald as a baby ostrich, walked with a limp, and couldn't get up from a chair without someone else's help. I resisted the urge to slap him on the spot. The experience was still too fresh, the wounds too raw. I deflected his questions with a sarcastic comment to mask how incensed I was that he'd presume I had manifested my own near-demise.

Years later, however, I began asking the same questions of myself. What *was* the purpose of having had a near-fatal illness? I began to make room for the possibility that I might, in some way, have chosen this experience, not on a conscious level, but perhaps on a soul level—the key word being *perhaps*. Could it be that my illness was an initiation? An expansion of my understanding of suffering, with the outgrowth of compassion? Or perhaps its purpose was to teach me how to be helped and loved and cared for by others. Or to offer a clean break from my old way of life, allowing me to move forward free from the burden of outmoded beliefs. I don't have the definitive answer, but choose instead to simply embrace the mystery of Life with a capital L.

Jeff prefers to take an existentialist's view of our shared experience. Even when I first met my husband and he was immersed in the world of business and technology, I could tell that underneath the starched button-down shirt and gray suit was a philosopher waiting patiently for release. Shortly after we moved in together, I noticed books by Nietzsche and Sartre and Kierkegaard appearing on his bedside table. He read them at night, for *fun*. Six years ago, when he began his doctoral studies in earnest, what was once a handful of philosophy books became an expansive home library. He befriended Hazel Barnes, a ninety-year-old retired philosophy professor, and the two of them spent hours together, sipping scotch and discussing existential concepts. At times, Jeff would launch into a philosophical soliloquy in my presence, and I, struggling to make sense of his academic terms and theories, would have to fight the urge to let my eyes glaze over and my mind wander. Once, I decided I'd had enough.

"Look," I said. "Pretend I'm a moron. Now, define existentialism for me in a simple way that I can actually understand."

"Okay," Jeff said. "It's about the personal responsibility that comes with absolute freedom. In other words, don't wait around for the promise of great things in the afterlife. Get off your ass and create the life you want *here and now*."

"You know what? I finally get it!" I said. "And in many ways, this whole preeclampsia thing has been one big lesson in exis-

... :ialism. It gave us permission to get off our asses and live the way we really wanted to."

"Exactly!" Jeff said.

And with that one conversation, I realized that my husband and I had even more in common than I'd thought. We're *both* existentialists, both willing to own the personal responsibility of creating the life we want. And yet we retain vastly different beliefs about matters of the spirit and have freely shared these differing perspectives with Clare, a budding philosopher in her own right.

Once, while strolling the aisles of Target, Clare, then six, asked, "Mom, why are we here?"

"I need to get a few things," I replied.

"No. I mean, why are we *here*?"

"Oh. What's the purpose of our lives?"

"Yes!"

"No one really knows for sure," I said. "People have lots of ideas, though."

"What do *you* think?"

"I think that maybe life is a big school and we come here to learn things, like how to create, or how to get along with others, or how to believe in ourselves. And because there are so many different classes to choose from, we might be learning different things than our friends are learning."

"Hmm," Clare said, turning this concept over in her mind. "That makes sense."

"You know how much you like school?"

"Yeah."

"Well, I think life is supposed to be like that too. Even if you don't like all the things the teacher makes you do or all the kids in your class, overall, it's supposed to be fun."

"Cool."

My daughter and I continue to share our evolving views about what our purpose is, why we came into being, and the possibility that there is no real death, only a passing away of the physical form from a soul that is eternal. We talk about my deceased father, Granddad Lee, with whom Clare feels a kinship despite never having met him. We talk about Spike, whose stiff body and blackened teeth my daughter asked to touch hours after our cancer-ridden poodle died peacefully in my arms when Clare was five. And recently, when Jeff's friend and mentor, Hazel, had died, and I told Clare about it during our drive to the grocery store, she asked me where I thought Hazel's spirit was now.

"I don't know for sure," I said, "But you know, Hazel didn't believe there was an afterlife."

"Well, won't *she* be surprised," Clare replied, not a trace of mockery in her voice.

It is these tender snippets of life with my daughter that often bring tears to my eyes in the unlikeliest of places. Last month, it happened as we sat facing one another in a grimy green vinyl booth at our favorite pizzeria, sharing a slice as an after-school snack, and the simplicity of the moment overwhelmed me. Watching her board the school bus each morning has made me teary on more than one occasion. And when she started a tickle fight in the back of a cab while accompanying me on a business trip back East, I found myself giggling and crying simultaneously. But nothing makes my chest tighten more than watching Clare reach out to the world—when she demands that I stop the car in the middle of running errands so she can share her "giving money" with yet another homeless person she's spotted on the curbside. She cried so hard after one such encounter that I drove around the block so she could give the same woman another $5 bill, this time from *my* wallet.

Did Clare arrive on the planet with this much compassion already stored in her being? Or did her experience of nearly suffocating at birth and then being taken from her parents for two months alter her, cracking her soul open wide to embrace the suffering of others, as it did for me?

During my travels and speaking, I've come across enough sadness and heartache to last a lifetime, stories from parents who've had to watch their children suffer or worse, die young. After a talk in New Jersey, the father of a two-year-old Down Syndrome boy told me his son had recently been diagnosed with leukemia. Tears filled his eyes as he said he'd gladly trade places with him if he could. In Ohio, I met a young girl named Caroline, who beamed with pride when the image of her wearing a tiara filled the projection screen behind me at a blood donor appreciation banquet. I shared Caroline's story with hundreds of people that day, told them how ongoing blood transfusions were an integral part of her cancer treatments. Her mother phoned me several years later seeking advice on how to become more active as an advocate for children's cancer research. She was doing this, she explained, to honor Caroline, who had died one month shy of her seventh birthday. There is almost a sense of guilt that washes over me each time I learn of another parent's loss, not only of a child, but of those simple moments of exquisite joy—the pizza slices, tickle fights, and jogs to catch the school bus—that will no longer be shared.

As my speaking engagements increased over the years, I found myself sliding into the precarious role of motivational speaker, with its temptation to put a positive spin on whatever life serves up, telling people what a gift my illness had been, how I wouldn't trade it for the world because so much good came from it. And perhaps I genuinely believed that. However, a year or so ago, when I again described my horrific experience—and by association, other people's horrific experiences—as a "blessing," I immediately heard my internal voice shout *What a load of crap!* It was as if my self-imposed obligation to whitewash all that sadness and hurt with a happily-ever-after veneer had been suddenly debunked, and I began to wonder why, for so long, I'd felt the need to treat life's heartbreaking losses with an upbeat bias. I stopped trying to explain : the suffering I encountered, stopped trying to force-fit it into some system of karma or divine will or goodness disguised as loss. Does someone who has never lost a child have the right to say *He's in a better place* or *Everything happens for a reason* to the mother who has just buried hers? Instead, I decided to simply sit with the suffering of others, allow it to touch that well of empathy within me, and then, if there was a way to help—and help was indeed wanted—I would. How dare I brush off the suffering of others by brushing off my own.

No, my experience of nearly dying was neither a gift nor was it a blessing.

But it was an *opportunity*. A huge, and not-to-be-repeated, opportunity for Jeff and me to survey the rubble that my illness left in its wake, to pick up each building block of our life together and examine its worth, then decide whether to keep it or not. Whether to rebuild the same life we had before or not.

Twelve-hour workdays in corporations that have no vested interest in our happiness or creative expression were the first to fall by the wayside. We immediately eliminated phrases like "someday we'll ..." from our vocabulary. We discarded outmoded notions that no longer fit our new perspective: that meaningful work must be postponed until there's enough of a bank account in place; that taking time to swim in the middle of a workday or to go for a daylong hike in the middle of the week is somehow irresponsible; or that moving to the south of France for a three-month sabbatical is not only impractical but impossible. All of these tenets that no longer served us we tossed without a second thought. And to fill the void of their departure, we increased our use of two words: *Why not?*

At times I get nervous about our future, but I remind myself that few things could present a greater challenge than what Jeff, Clare, and I have already faced with preeclampsia. And then I laugh, recalling what my friend Theresa, a two-time breast cancer survivor, said to her notoriously intimidating new boss: "You don't scare me. I've had chemo!"

On a cloudless summer day in 2007, I sit at a corner table on the terrace of Chez Serge Restaurant in Provence and lift my glass of *vin rouge* in a silent toast to the richness of life. *Why not,* indeed.

EPILOGUE

I STAND CENTER STAGE, completely at ease, and look out at the crowd. I've addressed more than 55,000 people in live audiences over the past six years, my largest venue holding more than 9,000 attendees. The turnout tonight is less than three hundred. I've given hundreds of radio, television, and newspaper interviews tied to my speaking tour, reaching an additional six million people. Tonight, there will be no media coverage.

I've spoken at fund-raisers and awareness events, conferences and banquets, typically as the keynote speaker, making people laugh and cry as I share stories related to the causes that are now an integral part of my life: volunteer blood donation, preeclampsia education and research, turning compassion into action. Tonight, I'm merely the emcee, and my job is to shepherd the luminaries of this event through their performances. Preparing to make my next introduction, I'm overcome with pride and giddy with joy.

"Ladies and gentlemen, from the third grade, please welcome Clare Larsen!"

With the sound of applause in the background, I watch my eight-year-old daughter gulp hard, as if to swallow her nervousness, and make her way from behind the stage curtain toward the worn upright piano. She keeps her gaze focused on the destination, with not even a fleeting glimpse at the audience. The first two fingers on each hand are tightly crossed, Clare's customary behavior when she wants to ensure that something goes her way. On more than one occasion I've quietly observed this finger-crossing habit as she approached me with a special request. *Can Poet sleep over? Can we go to the movies? Can we get a dachshund?* Who am I to dispute the efficacy of this simple gesture of hers? Did we not adopt a ten-year-old wiener dog just last month?

Clare is wearing her favorite special-occasion outfit: the velvet jumpsuit, crimson on top and black on the bottom, with sparkly rhinestones across the chest. A black velvet headband adorns her long hair and helps disguise the wireless microphone headset. Around her neck is the silver heart-shaped necklace I received as a gift at a speaking engagement two years ago. And on her feet, the black go-go boots that Santa brought her this year, though I suspect she knows they came from me.

She sits on the piano bench and sets her sheet music above the keyboard, allowing herself one quick glance toward my mother in the third row and briefly smiling in recognition. I'm sure the videographer in the back of the gymnasium shares my sense of delight because it's my husband who mans the camera.

Jeff and I have spent the past three weeks immersed in auditions and rehearsals for the elementary school's annual talent show. As the event's coproducers, we've been working with more than 140 kids, kindergarteners through fifth graders, and it has been utterly exhausting. It has also been priceless, and more gratifying than I imagined, to watch their individual acts come together, their confidence build—not the least of which our daughter's.

The clapping subsides, as does the shuffling of feet and clearing of throats, and for a moment there is silence. I implore unseen forces to make the next several minutes go well for Clare. It's not the bragging rights of a perfect performance that I seek, but the desire for my child to thoroughly enjoy the expression of her creative self, to share her beautiful soul with the world. Then Clare begins singing and playing "Falling Slowly" from the movie *Once*, which I allowed her to see despite its R rating. She chose this piece for the talent show shortly after we watched it win an Oscar last year during our annual mother-daughter Academy Awards party. I found the lyrics online and downloaded them for her, and I remember being struck by the words when I first read them, how they reflected my feelings about Clare long before I was pregnant.

I don't know you,
But I want you
All the more for that.

The significance of this moment—Clare at the piano, Mom in the audience, Jeff at the back of the room, me backstage—and what we've collectively survived to get here, shakes me to the core. I fan my eyes with my note cards to keep the tears at bay, but the love I feel for my daughter overwhelms me with emotion. To me, her voice sounds like that of an angel. And why wouldn't it? She is, after all, named for one.

What was it about the offbeat but kindhearted Clarence Oddbody from my favorite movie that enticed me to make him my daughter's namesake? Was there some unconscious knowledge that, just as Clarence did for George Bailey, Clare would make me appreciate all the perfect imperfections of my life? Help me better understand the value of my very existence? I've seen *It's a Wonderful Life* more than twenty-five times and can recite much of the dialogue by heart. Yet without fail, I cry unabashedly every time George leans over that bridge—head bowed, hands clasped, tears streaming down his face—and implores his guardian angel, Clarence, to let him live again.

Take this sinking boat
And point it home,
We've still got time.

Clare first watched *It's a Wonderful Life* with me when she was six, and she too cried at this same point in the movie, as if she intrinsically understood its parallel to our own lives. We were sharing a bowl of onion dip, but once George was on that bridge the potato chip in Clare's hand stopped in midair and never made it to the dip bowl, her focus on the movie so intense. George reached in his pocket and pulled out his daughter's rose petals, proof that his wish to live again had just been granted. "Zuzu's petals!" he exclaimed, his facial expression a mix of wonder and delight.

Crying, Clare left her beanbag chair and joined me in mine. I wrapped her in my arms and held her close as George ran through the snow-covered streets of downtown Bedford Falls, euphoric that he'd been given a second chance. Neither she nor I said a word until George was back in his living room surrounded by a lifetime of friends, and he opened the front cover of *Tom Sawyer*, which Clarence had left as a farewell gift.

"What does it say?" Clare asked.

"*Dear George: Remember, no man is a failure who has friends,*" I said, swallowing hard.

George looked to the heavens and winked in acknowledgment to his angel. And I gave mine a squeeze.

"I'm really glad Dad brought us roses that time," Clare said.

My daughter has attended many of my speaking events, and it is this detail of our shared story that stands out most for her. She has heard me refer to the roses as providence, a deliberate prompting from unknown forces. She has heard Jeff refer to it as chance, a benevolent yet random occurrence. What she has *not* yet heard is a detail I myself learned years after her birth, when a nurse practitioner who'd cared for Clare helped me decipher her medical record. According to the "cord gas reading" taken at the time of her delivery, Clare had perhaps fifteen more minutes before she would've died in utero, before she would've become another heartbreaking statistic of fetal mortality due to preeclampsia. By taking the time to bring me roses that afternoon Jeff saved Clare's life, and perhaps mine as well. Whether by divine intervention or dumb luck, it matters not.

Raise your hopeful voice
You have a choice
You'll make it now.

I used to think I had a pretty wonderful life. And then I got sick. And I saw no way home. And I wanted to die. Then a miracle happened. Something within me shifted and I wanted to live. In the worst way, I wanted to live again. Surrounded by "angels" who helped me—nurses, doctors, blood donors, family, friends, Jeff, and later, Clare—I became the George Bailey of my own life.

Not every aspect of my story, however, wrapped up with a tidy Hollywood ending the way it did in the movie. Turns out the publishing colleague who amiably chided me for setting out to do a marathon so soon after my illness was right. It *was* a stupid idea. Aside from the positive impact on my psyche, running that race set my physical recovery back by years and caused permanent damage to my joints. Shortly after coming home from New York in 2001, my right shoulder froze and continues to be frozen eight years later despite tens of thousands of dollars spent on treatments not covered by our deficient health insurance policy. My knees, ankles, and feet are chronically arthritic, at times aching unmercifully. Since my first bowel obstruction, I've had six more. And at age forty-seven, I feel as though I possess the body of a seventy-five-year-old.

There were also several not-so-wonderful-life outcomes for my personal support team, those intricately involved in my survival. Tim and Dede's life together disintegrated shortly after they both worked so hard to help Jeff and me retain ours. They're now divorced. Val's MS advanced, and for the past four years she's been confined to an electric wheelchair, her right arm the only functioning limb on her body. And my stepdad was diagnosed with malignant mesothelioma—cancer caused by asbestos—as he was preparing to leave on one of his coveted weeklong bike trips. Seven months later he was dead.

Perhaps the point is not to judge life as being *either* cruel or wonderful, a veil of tears or a bowl of cherries. Perhaps it's about accepting that suffering and joy co-exist and embracing both, even honoring the role that each plays in the rich tapestry of our lives, the balance they offer. While no one denies the benefit of joy, there are those who wish to hide from its less popular counterpart. Yet doesn't the suffering of others offer the opportunity for each of us to step up and be someone's angel? And, even more challenging for many of us, doesn't our *own* suffering teach us how to allow others to be *our* angels, to open our hearts to the compassion that others have to give?

Halfway through *It's a Wonderful Life*, when Clarence sees that George has lost hope and is about to kill himself, he leaps from the bridge into the same frozen river that George is eyeing. George, now refocused on someone else's problems, plunges in after Clarence and his perspective shifts from despair to hope, from *needing* an angel to *being* an angel.

"I knew if I were drowning, you'd try to save me," Clarence tells him later. "And that's how *I* saved *you*."

We've come to Clare's big finish, the final chorus followed by the fading out of the piano. I'm sure she's feeling both relief and exhilaration right now because she knows she made it. Though for different reasons, I feel the same way.

Falling slowly
Sing your melody,
I'll sing along.

I dry my eyes and prepare for the next act.

ACKNOWLEDGMENTS

Writing a book is no easy task, especially if you're dead. So first and foremost, a big shout-out to all blood donors. Without your selfless acts of kindness, millions of us—myself included—wouldn't be here to tell our stories. Heartfelt thanks to the more than two hundred strangers who shared their blood with me, including Raul Alfaro, Nick Barbarotto, Roger Capilos, Charles Fairbrother, Craig Friske, Louise Gaither, Deborah Higgins, Matt Lawler, George Menzoian, Colin Peacock, Herman Santos, Athena Schmitz, Keith Smith, Karl Sutphin, John Sweeney, Adam Thaler, Rick Weil, Kristen Wells, Stephen Westrick, and James Willis. Meeting you in person remains one of the highlights of my life.

Gallons of gratitude go to the good people at Blood Centers of the Pacific and United Blood Services, two fine organizations that did whatever it took to give a new mom a second chance. Lisa Bloch, Nora Hirschler, Deb Verkouw, and Angela Woon were among the first blood bankers I'd ever met. Your kindness and encouragement made me want to do everything possible to help the cause.

Big hugs go to Carol Abrahams, John Alexander, Peter Chordas, Denise Harrington, Margaret Haytaian, Susan Hills, Les Kiley-Smith, Suzanne Reno, Carol Snyder, and Susan Warren, all of whom bear out my theory that nurses are nothing short of angels in comfy shoes. You each possess the perfect blend of knowledge to heal the body and nurturing to heal the soul.

Kudos to the docs whose expertise and teamwork somehow did the trick (with apologies for any expletives I may have hurled at you), in particular Michael Borah, Chris Brown, Michael Fahmy, Chris Freise, Laurie Green, Ilyas Iliya, Michael Katz, Elliot Main, Lisa Moy, Anne O'Duffy, Bob Osorio, Carl Otto, Jenta Shen, Patricia St. Clare, Steve Steady, Bertrand Tuan, Michael Valan, and Adil Wakil. Bob, if your bedside manner could be bottled and sold, I'm certain there would be a dramatic decrease in medical liability lawsuits overnight.

Much appreciation to all the other nurses, doctors, and other specialists from California Pacific Medical Center—more than one hundred forty total—whose skills helped me defy the odds: C. Allmon-Carroll, Elizabeth Anderson, Edna Arenal, Fareed Asfour, Guialyn Baldoza, Jamil Brewster, Rebecca Brown, Kathleen Capp, Cynthia Casey, Mary Jane Cerzo, Theresa Chu, Ruben Clay, Regina Connell, Carol Conrardy, Peri Corsiglia, Thomas Cromwell, Ann Marie Dalisay, Carol Ann D'Amico, Frank Delen, Karen Devaney, Cheryl Duffy, James Durrett, Amrita Dutta-Choudhury, Christina Eardley, Ronald Elkin, Bryan Ellis, Davene Fernandez, Joi Fernelius, Rafael Fletes, Chris Foster, Jeffrey Fung, Margo Gasparino, Robert Gish, Joanne Goettshe, S. Gonzales, Alex Goodman, Sharon Gross, Victoria Gross, Michelle Hamre, Nanette Hinojales, Pat Hodges, Peter Hosseinpour, Kun Huang, Anna Huh, Thomas Jackson, Adrianne Jaski, Barbara Jones, N. Kamangar, Mark Kasselik, Maryam Khotani, Oksook Kim, Barbara King, Nympha Kinsolving, Helen Kosik, Julia Kringen, Ying Kuan, Belinda Kwan, Paula Landdeck, Hoa Le, Katie Lee, Susie Lim, Mee Mee Lin, Margaret Litawa, Gala Li-Wong, Stephen Lockhart,

Amy Logsdon, Celeste Louis, Jocelyn Luna, Cindy Lux, Diane Magallanes, Mina Mai, Kevin Marshall, Krystyna Marvinov, Myron Marx, Adam Mason, Kristin McCarten, Dana McClure, Nancy McGrath-Klein, Clair McNamara, Leland Monagle, Graciela Montes, Michelle Murray, Byron Nguyen, Gina Nguyen, Jodi Oronsky, Ann Marie O'Sullivan, Basilisa Pagtakhan, Richard Park, J. Phattanagosai, Sue Priddy, Victor Prokopov, Jennifer Quaglia, Lori Quan, Pat Radosevich, Minerva Ramos, Aaron Rang, John Riordan, Janice Roth, Soudip Ted Saha, Prerana Sangani, Sally Scagel, Margaret Schmidt, James Schwanke, Loretta Seeley, Monica Stratton, Susan Tanaka, Betty Tang, Veronica Ton, Barbara Torio, Brenda Tune, Keith Umezawa, Sharon Urbiztondo, Stephanie Vaccaro, Lisa Vipiana, Steven Vitcov, Jon Wack, Barbara Walsh, Janet Walsh, Jeff Wang, Rae Wang, Linda Weaver, Anne Wegener, Dianne Weyna, Victoria Wiley, Debbie Williams, Heather Wilson, Amy Wiluz, Lee Wolfer, Cheon Yee, Betty Yip, and Margaret Zimmerman. Wow, it truly takes a village, doesn't it?

Dusa Rammessirsingh, you are one of the finest energy healers on this planet. I still don't understand it all, but I know you played an instrumental role in my care in the ICU. Others from the complementary healing professions who helped during my hospitalization include Phil Cullinan, Laurie Garrett, and Roberta Leigh. Kudos to each of you for integrating the unconventional into mainstream medicine.

Loving noogies to my family members, who came from all corners of the country to help me pull through (or secure dibs on my bike if I didn't): Mom and John (we miss you, Pa), Bev and Rud Hoag, Stephanie Myers, Karen Scalzi, Val and Mark Taylor, Tim Ward (aka Uncle Buffalo Head), and Dede Ward, as well as my three gal pals who've since been adopted into the family: Sabra Horne, Pam Hussey, and Liz Rockhold. Um, sorry about all that. And at Karen's suggestion, the next time I "want attention," I promise to simply pick up the phone and call.

Recovery kudos to Robin Claire, Terry Hambrick, Sam Iannetta, Inge Moorby, Elizabeth North, Bill Shiovitz, and Brian Thelen. Surviving was one thing. But thriving took a team of coaches, and each of you played a significant role in rebuilding my body.

Deepest appreciation to Bill Nielsen, who transformed my grassroots give-back effort into a national program. Many thanks to others at Johnson & Johnson who also helped along the way: Isabelle Barber, Sarah Colamarino, Jeff Colella, Roy Davis, Russ Deyo, Carol Dobrovolski, Kathy Ducsak, Linda Gallo, Rob Halper, Ray Jordan, Nancy Lewin, Susan Odenthal, Theresa Ragozine, Mary Richardson, Tom Sullivan, Dave Swearingen, and Bill Weldon. Boy, you weren't kidding when you said that having a baby changes everything.

Gratitude to those who continue to seek answers and educate others about preeclampsia, including Preeclampsia Foundation founders Anne Garrett Addison and Tom Easterling, as well as Ananth Karumanchi, Jaime and Joe Nolan, Baha Sibai, Jill and Jeff Siegel, Eleni Tsigas, John and Brenda Warner, and all my PE sisters who've shared their stories with me for various advocacy projects. Together, I know we can improve pregnancy outcomes in the future for our daughters, granddaughters, and all expectant moms around the world.

Blessings to Jenny Eller and Shelly Bridgewater—two special young women whose stories ended too soon. You both continue to inspire me daily.

Sincere appreciation goes to the In The Telling Press publishing team: Joe Fierst, Loretta Goodenbour, Gary Head, Kathie

Head, Patty Hodgins, Sande Johnson, and Alice Levine. Together, you were finally able to yank that manuscript from my grip and turn it into a book, thereby giving my life back to me a second time.

Endless gratitude to those author-teachers who taught me to forget the business of writing and enjoy the craft of storytelling: Barbara Abercrombie, Shari Caudron, Ann Hood, and Abigail Thomas. May your words continue to inspire others as they have me.

Big hugs to my story-shaping, word-chopping, ever supportive TH4: Denise Clemen, Jamie Marshall, and Ken Olsen. At the risk of eliciting a Cliché Alert, you are the wind beneath my writing wings. I could easily give you "two pages" on how grateful I am to Abby and the Tin House Summer Writers Workshop for connecting us.

I am in awe of the love and encouragement I received from my best friend, life partner, and #1 honey-bunny, Jeff. You knew when to send me away to write, when to laugh or cry as I read early drafts aloud, and when to make me set it all aside to curl up with you and Clare for a bowl of onion dip and a stupid humor movie. You are, and will remain, my OTL.

And finally, "leaf-wise" hugs to my Clare Bear, who is the embodiment of compassion in action. You continue to inspire me to be my best—for you, for our little family, for the world. With you, Dad, Ghee, Gigs, Duke, and Stinky Boy Jack by my side, it truly is a wonderful life.

ABOUT THE AUTHOR

Lauren Ward Larsen is the chief ambassador of the Foundation for America's Blood Centers, based in Washington, D.C. She is also an international speaker and advocate for preeclampsia research and awareness, volunteer blood donation, and clean water initiatives in Sudan. For all of her grassroots efforts to promote blood donation, Larsen was awarded the 2001 Larry Frederick Award from America's Blood Centers. She was also the recipient of the 2006 Outstanding Achievement Award presented by the American Association of Blood Banks. She holds a B.A. from the University of Arizona and an M.B.A. from U.C.L.A. Lauren, her husband Jeff, and daughter Clare live in Boulder, Colorado, where they laugh often and take nothing for granted.

To contact Lauren Ward Larsen about her work, speaking availability, or humanitarian initiatives (or to simply gawk at some nasty photos from the intensive care unit), please visit:

www.laurenwardlarsen.com

For more information about bulk-order discounts for *Zuzu's Petals,* please contact:

zuzuspetals@inthetelling.com

For more information about volunteer blood donation, please visit one of the sites below:

www.americasblood.org
www.redcrossblood.org
www.aabb.org

For more information about preeclampsia and HELLP Syndrome, please visit:

www.preeclampsia.org

In The Telling Press is a social enterprise publisher committed to making a difference while making a profit. Together, the author and the publisher commit to donating at least ten percent of the selling price of each publication to related charitable causes. Donations from *Zuzu's Petals* will support global efforts to provide a safe and adequate blood supply, preeclampsia research and education, nursing scholarships, and/or clean water initiatives in Sudan.